PAIN MANAGEMENT – RESEARCH AND TECHNOLOGY

CHRONIC PAIN

PREVALENCE, MANAGEMENT AND OUTCOMES

PAIN MANAGEMENT – RESEARCH AND TECHNOLOGY

Additional books and e-books in this series can be found on Nova's website under the Series tab.

PAIN MANAGEMENT – RESEARCH AND TECHNOLOGY

CHRONIC PAIN

PREVALENCE, MANAGEMENT AND OUTCOMES

STEFAN FRIEDMAN
EDITOR

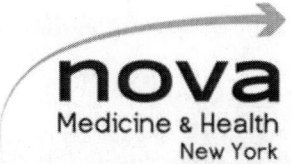

Copyright © 2019 by Nova Science Publishers, Inc.

All rights reserved. No part of this book may be reproduced, stored in a retrieval system or transmitted in any form or by any means: electronic, electrostatic, magnetic, tape, mechanical photocopying, recording or otherwise without the written permission of the Publisher.

We have partnered with Copyright Clearance Center to make it easy for you to obtain permissions to reuse content from this publication. Simply navigate to this publication's page on Nova's website and locate the "Get Permission" button below the title description. This button is linked directly to the title's permission page on copyright.com. Alternatively, you can visit copyright.com and search by title, ISBN, or ISSN.

For further questions about using the service on copyright.com, please contact:
Copyright Clearance Center
Phone: +1-(978) 750-8400   Fax: +1-(978) 750-4470   E-mail: info@copyright.com

NOTICE TO THE READER

The Publisher has taken reasonable care in the preparation of this book, but makes no expressed or implied warranty of any kind and assumes no responsibility for any errors or omissions. No liability is assumed for incidental or consequential damages in connection with or arising out of information contained in this book. The Publisher shall not be liable for any special, consequential, or exemplary damages resulting, in whole or in part, from the readers' use of, or reliance upon, this material. Any parts of this book based on government reports are so indicated and copyright is claimed for those parts to the extent applicable to compilations of such works.

Independent verification should be sought for any data, advice or recommendations contained in this book. In addition, no responsibility is assumed by the Publisher for any injury and/or damage to persons or property arising from any methods, products, instructions, ideas or otherwise contained in this publication.

This publication is designed to provide accurate and authoritative information with regard to the subject matter covered herein. It is sold with the clear understanding that the Publisher is not engaged in rendering legal or any other professional services. If legal or any other expert assistance is required, the services of a competent person should be sought. FROM A DECLARATION OF PARTICIPANTS JOINTLY ADOPTED BY A COMMITTEE OF THE AMERICAN BAR ASSOCIATION AND A COMMITTEE OF PUBLISHERS.

Additional color graphics may be available in the e-book version of this book.

Library of Congress Cataloging-in-Publication Data

ISBN: 978-1-53616-296-7
Library of Congress Control Number:2019950412

Published by Nova Science Publishers, Inc. † New York

CONTENTS

Preface vii

Chapter 1 Managing Chronic Pain: Using Practical Brief
Psychological and Hypnotic Interventions 1
Ann Williamson

Chapter 2 The Journey to Coping:
A Grounded Theory of Pain Coping amongst
Maltese Chronic Pain Sufferers 27
Pamela Portelli and Clare Eldred

Chapter 3 Self-Empowerment, Self-Efficacy and
Mindfulness: Does Multidisciplinary
Pain Therapy Inhibit or Support? 59
Michael Hartmann and Jutta Kirchner

Chapter 4 Insurers Save While Patients Pay:
The Redistribution of Medication Costs
Following Enrollment in a State-Legal Medical
Cannabis Program 73
*Sarah S. Stith, Jacob M. Vigil, Ian Adams
and Anthony P. Reeve*

Index 99

Related Nova Publications 105

PREFACE

In the opening chapter of Chronic Pain: Prevalence, Management and Outcomes, the authors examine how the health care professional might psychologically approach the management of chronic pain. The nocebo effect of some communications will be highlighted, as well as ways to utilise the patient's internal resources to reduce emotional distress.

Following this, a study exploring pain coping mechanisms amongst Maltese chronic pain patients is presented. Semi-structured interviews were conducted with 21 participants, and findings derived from a grounded theory methodology revealed that Maltese often display reluctance to rely on pharmacological therapies.

The authors address the need for pain treatment, the reduced interference of interventional pain management, the increase of patient self-efficacy, and methods of acceptance for some chronic pain.

The closing chapter analyzes 3,434 scheduled prescription drug records for 94 chronic back pain patients from a single clinic, comparing 52 patients enrolled in the New Mexico Medical Cannabis Program with 42 non-enrolled patients over a 24 month period.

Chapter 1 - Working as a GP (family doctor) for over thirty years, having to manage patients with chronic pain was not uncommon. These patients present a complex problem that encompasses feelings of loss and distress as well as a change of identity or role, alongside pain symptoms. Although chemical analgesia plays an important part in the management of these patients' pain, it does not address the psychological and emotional aspects and sometimes leads to problems with side effects, addiction or tolerance. This chapter examines how the health care professional might approach the management of chronic pain, using psychological approaches. The nocebo effect of some communications will be highlighted and ways of giving a more positive communication demonstrated. Ways to utilise the patient's internal resources and imagination to reduce emotional distress will be discussed. Hypnosis and imagery have been shown to have an effect not only on the psychological distress associated with chronic pain but also to have an effect on the experienced intensity of the pain. Simple techniques that can be taught to patients such as self-hypnosis and use of imagery will be presented. There is increasing evidence for the effectiveness of hypnosis in the management of pain and neuroscience evidence is throwing light on the mechanisms involved.

Chapter 2 - This chapter comprises a study exploring pain coping mechanisms amongst Maltese chronic pain patients. Semi structured interviews were conducted with 21 participants. Findings derived from a grounded theory methodology revealed that Maltese often display a seeming reluctance to rely on pharmacological therapies, relying on a number of self-taught/sought strategies. The journey to coping is not an easy one, with some participants engaging in relentless struggles to eliminate pain. The inability to achieve control often leads to a sense of disconnectedness from the external world. Sometimes, death by suicide is perceived as the only solution, albeit an unacceptable one. Although religion may be a protective factor against suicide, it also seemed a major impediment because participants perceived suicide as sinful in the eyes of God. On the other hand, effective self-preservation strategies can foster a sense of acceptance. The importance of taking into account the religious and cultural dimension in the pain experience was identified.

Chapter 3 - Objectives: Today's pain management ought to be executed in a multidisciplinary and - even better - an interdisciplinary setting. Unfortunately, due to various types of discourse and different beliefs, this may lead to non-acceptance of the other party's competence and might even be judged as an offence to one's own practice. To achieve an increase in the mutual appreciation of the somatic and the psychological perspective we address:

- the imperative need of pain-treatment for the patient who is in distress:
- the reduced interference of interventional pain management with the patient's self-empowerment compared to medical therapy with long-lasting pharmaceuticals;
- the increase of self-efficacy once the patient's "active" mode is (re-)installed; and
- methods of accepting some chronic pain using tools to remove the focus on pain from the patient's attention.

Methods: In order to also consider pain as an expression of suffering, which is an integral part of life, we have consulted philosophical sources. In order to evaluate long-term, and in particular drug therapy, pain-specific self-efficacy and mindfulness techniques, we conducted a database search (pubmed). Results: Chronic pain and suffering have to be discussed not in a utilitarian framework but in a phenomenological context inspired by Schopenhauer, Wittgenstein, Jaspers, van Buitendijk, Scheler and Merleau-Ponty. There is an imperative need for pain-treatment for the patient who is in distress. No literature could be identified regarding whether or not interventional pain management implies reduced interference with patients' self-empowerment compared to medical therapy with long-lasting pharmaceuticals. Studies on self-efficacy and those on methods of accepting some chronic pain will be discussed. Discussion: Chronic pain, as all suffering, develops from being essential to being existential. To a certain extent, it is a contingent part of life, and it might even be meaningful. A multidisciplinary team therapy should generally be targeted at lowering the pain level to create valences for the patients, to subsequently enable them to take control again.

Chapter 4 - State-level analyses have found prescription cost savings associated with the legalization of medical cannabis, yet little is known about how patient-level shifts in conventional medication use lead to aggregate cost savings and how they compare to medical cannabis costs. We analyze 3,434 scheduled prescription drug records for 94 chronic back pain patients from a single clinic, comparing 52 patients enrolled in the New Mexico Medical Cannabis Program (MCP) with 42 non-enrolled patients over a 24-month period. We calculate adjusted costs to insurers and patients based on average wholesale prices, dispensing fees, and patient copays and use a difference-in-differences fixed effects panel regression approach to study the association between MCP enrollment and conventional prescription drug costs. Cannabis costs are based on patient survey responses. Relative to pre-enrollment or our comparison group, MCP-enrolled patients' conventional prescriptions cost almost $200 less to insurers per month and $30 less out-of-pocket to patients at 18 months post-enrollment. With monthly medical cannabis costs of $141 (SD=$91), patients faced higher out-of-pocket costs than they did prior to enrollment in the MCP, suggesting a strong preference for cannabis. From a total cost perspective, combined insurer and patient cost savings on conventional prescriptions outweigh the costs of medical cannabis after 11 months post-enrollment in the MCP.

In: Chronic Pain
Editor: Stefan Friedman

ISBN: 978-1-53616-296-7
© 2019 Nova Science Publishers, Inc.

Chapter 1

MANAGING CHRONIC PAIN: USING PRACTICAL BRIEF PSYCHOLOGICAL AND HYPNOTIC INTERVENTIONS

*Ann Williamson**
Mossley, Manchester, UK

ABSTRACT

Working as a GP (family doctor) for over thirty years, having to manage patients with chronic pain was not uncommon. These patients present a complex problem that encompasses feelings of loss and distress as well as a change of identity or role, alongside pain symptoms. Although chemical analgesia plays an important part in the management of these patients' pain, it does not address the psychological and emotional aspects and sometimes leads to problems with side effects, addiction or tolerance. This chapter examines how the health care professional might approach the management of chronic pain, using psychological approaches. The nocebo effect of some communications will be highlighted and ways of giving a more positive communication demonstrated. Ways to utilise the patient's internal resources and imagination to reduce emotional distress will be

---

* Corresponding Author's E-mail: ann@annwilliamson.co.uk.

discussed. Hypnosis and imagery have been shown to have an effect not only on the psychological distress associated with chronic pain but also to have an effect on the experienced intensity of the pain. Simple techniques that can be taught to patients such as self-hypnosis and use of imagery will be presented. There is increasing evidence for the effectiveness of hypnosis in the management of pain and neuroscience evidence is throwing light on the mechanisms involved.

Keywords: chronic pain, anxiety, depression, hypnosis, imagery, positive suggestion

INTRODUCTION

Chronic pain is usually defined as pain present for more than three months and studies have shown that it affects between a third and a half of the UK population, and has an increasing prevalence with age (Fayaz et al. 2016). We know that the sensation of pain is not merely a simple response to tissue damage but that a whole neuromatrix is activated, not only by sensory input, but also affected by cultural influence, past experience and emotional state. So, far from being a passive recipient of information about actual or potential damage, neurones in the brain and spinal cord actively process and modulate the sensory information received from the periphery. In acute contexts the sensation of pain can be seen as a warning message, alerting us to avoid further possible damage. Chronic pain may arise following an initial injury, often musculoskeletal, such as back strain or be associated with ongoing illness, such as cancer. The pain neuromatrix is activated even though the warning function of the message is no longer required. Chronic pain may also have no obvious 'physical' cause but because it may have emotional and psychological underpinnings does not mean that the patient is not experiencing pain in just the same way as someone with an obvious injury, such as a fractured femur. It has also been shown that those with chronic pain have (or develop) a lowered threshold of reaction to noxious stimuli (Moseley 2003) so that their pain neuromatrix activates even sooner than normal. It is as if their smoke alarm activates when the toast is burning rather than when the kitchen is burning down.

Chronic pain also often leads to a loss of function and a reduction in activity and if these changes persist, they often have an adverse effect on the patient's emotional health. Muscle strength and balance may deteriorate due to lack of use. Stress relieving activities such as going to the gym, swimming, or walking may be reduced, with a subsequent rise in stress, anxiety and depression. This, as well as the chronic pain itself, may impact on sleep patterns giving rise to disturbed nights and daytime fatigue. Insufficient sleep is also associated with more snacking and obesity (Chaput 2014). Depression is often associated with chronic pain conditions (Bair 2003) as a reaction to the loss of physical health and there is a reciprocal effect of emotional distress on the perceived sensations of pain (Bushnell et al. 2013; Fishbain et al. 1997). This may especially be true of those with cancer pain, where patients may also be battling to come to terms with their own mortality and their feelings of lack of control over their own bodies, as they undergo procedures and chemotherapy.

Sometimes patients tend to define themselves through their chronic pain, taking it on at the level of identity rather than something that they are experiencing. This is a complex issue. Sometimes the 'illness' role of chronic pain can have consequences, such that the patient is unwilling, at an unconscious level, to relinquish that role. It may give them status or allow them to withdraw from activities or social events they are reluctant to participate in, so that even if consciously they want to be pain free, consideration needs to be given to these underlying unconscious elements for a successful outcome. If they no longer have their pain, all the adaptations that they have made in their life, physically, psychologically, and in their relationships have to be rethought. There is also the thought that if they could 'get rid' of their pain why hadn't they done so before? This is where educating the patient about the pain neuromatrix and the bio-psycho-social aspects of pain is so important.

Chemical analgesia has an important part to play in the management of chronic pain but alongside psycho-education and strategies for self-management. Side effects are common and increasing tolerance may lead to difficulty in obtaining effective relief.

Unfortunately, it may often be impossible for someone with chronic pain to become pain free but they can learn to manage their pain so that it no longer controls every aspect of their lives. Alongside learning to manage physical exercise and activities to the best of their ability, patients can be encouraged to learn ways to manage their emotional states and focus on what they want to achieve rather than focusing on their pain.

COMMUNICATION

Patients often find difficulty in accepting uncertainty and may feel better if they have a diagnosis or label for their symptoms. How this diagnosis is conveyed may have an important impact on the patient's experience. When a patient is in shock or feeling extremely anxious, anything they see or hear is communication, even if it is not directed at them. Also, if there are two interpretations of that communication, they will always choose the more negative.

Patients often still believe Descartes model of pain, relating pain directly to tissue damage and that the amount of pain equates to amount of physical damage they have. They need to be educated regarding the complexity of the pain neuromatrix and that even if no medical cause can be elicited their pain experience is not 'imaginary'. Ordering endless investigations is unproductive especially as a negative result does not provide re-assurance to the anxious patient (Petrie et al. 2007) but merely confirms that 'the doctor hasn't found the cause yet.' Equally some patients may have significant damage yet experience little in the way of discomfort.

It could be said that we have two ways of processing; a cognitive/rational processing system which could be seen as analogous to our left-brain or left cerebral hemisphere functioning, or conscious mind, and our sensory/imaginal processing system that is more right-brained or right cerebral hemisphere functioning, and more analogous to our unconscious processing (Brann 2012, 98-99). We know that simply knowing something intellectually does not always affect emotions. Think of the spider phobic who feels terror at the sight of a tiny eight-legged insect – they usually find it almost impossible to rationalise the fear away, even though they know that they are many times more powerful and could, physically, easily squash the spider under their shoe. However, working with metaphor and imagery can have a profound effect on how people feel and studies have shown that what is visualised in hypnosis activates similar areas of the brain as the real thing (Kosslyn et al. 2000).

Hypnosis has been defined as "A social interaction in which one person, designated the subject, responds to suggestions offered by another person, designated the hypnotist, for experiences involving alterations in perception, memory and voluntary action" (Kilstrom 1985).

Hypnosis could be seen as a descriptive label for a change from external to internal focus, from our external environment to our internal feelings and imagery. It requires a focus of attention, often on breathing and is often followed by suggestions of progressive muscular relaxation. This internally focused or meditative state decreases the patient's arousal response and allows suggestions to be more strongly accepted than in the 'normal' waking state. Suggestions may be given verbally or by using imagery, as will be described later.

Hypnosis has been used to treat every type of pain condition over centuries and across cultures (Pintar and Lynn, 2008) and can be an extremely effective treatment for both acute and chronic pain. It is one of the most well researched areas in clinical hypnosis.

A patient experiencing high levels of anxiety will already be in a hypnotic type state, functioning at an emotional rather than an intellectual, rational level, so words are often taken very literally. Communications such as describing a degenerative spine as 'crumbling' generates an image in the patient's mind that suggests a continuous on-going process that will always be painful. Equally using terms such as 'This won't hurt' imply that it will, as the unconscious mind does not compute negatives. In order to not think about something, you have to have thought about it first. Unfortunately, many healthcare professionals are not careful about the words they use, and even now are still taught to say 'Just a sharp scratch' when giving an injection or taking blood (Richter et al. 2010). The patient experience would be much better if they were told 'I am going to give you your injection/take your blood test now so, as I do that, I wonder if you could tell me...' Alternatively changing the patient's focus of attention by engaging them in a task such as counting how many items they can see in a picture on the wall can be helpful. Engaging the patient's imagination, as will be described later, to take them to somewhere of their choice "where nothing we do here need bother you at all" can be extremely effective.

The way a diagnosis of a chronic pain condition is given may have long-lasting effects. Although a 'label' such as Fibromyalgia or Chronic Fatigue Syndrome may reassure the patient that they are being taken seriously it is crucial that they do not become defined by their label – all patients need to understand that their pain is multi-factorial and that they are far more than the label given to their particular cluster of symptoms. What the patient imagines may be very far from the idea that the healthcare professional wished to convey.

> One patient came to see me with severe depression two years after she had received a diagnosis of multiple sclerosis. Her physical symptoms were unchanged over this time but the image she had 'seen' when told her diagnosis was of herself in a wheelchair, because one of her friends had the severe fulminating type of the condition. Once she had realised this link, she was able to accept that she had a much milder form of the disease and her depression gradually lifted.

To tell an anxious patient that they will have to learn to live with their pain implies that nothing can be done and that their pain will last until they die....

USING HYPNOSIS TO SET GOALS

Patients need to understand that they are more than their pain and that their pain is not what defines them as a person. This psychoeducation needs to be done once rapport has been obtained; each consultation is different and the clinician needs to balance acknowledgement of the current state of the patient, both physically and emotionally, with the goals that need to be achieved. Visualisation of having achieved the goal, whatever it is, whilst in a focused hypnotic state can be very helpful, boosting motivation. It is important to ensure that the patient understands what degree of exercise is useful, rather than deleterious to their condition. If management, rather than cure, is the likely outcome then it is crucial to focus the patient's attention on what they can do to help themselves and to give them small goals to work towards. Working with physiotherapy whilst the patient relaxes in hypnosis can be very effective (Lebon et al. 2017).

Closing the eyes, taking three deep breaths, breathing in calmness either as a feeling, a colour, or both, can serve as a quick way to focus internally. One then suggests that the patient imagines themselves having achieved their goal and then 'steps into' that image so that they can feel how it might be, say something internally such as 'I know I can do this' or 'This is the way to go' (or whatever is appropriate for them). They then open their eyes and then repeat the exercise four or five times, opening their eyes in between each cycle.

This can aid motivation and be a very useful exercise for patients to repeat daily. By using imagery in an associated way (stepping into the image) it connects the patient more strongly with what they are wanting to achieve or feel. It can also be used with good effect to help with anxiety provoking situations where the goal image would be dealing calmly with the situation. Anxiety management will be discussed further on, together with ways that imagery can be used to manage feelings.

Hypnotic approaches for pain relief typically take three forms: Direct suggestion for symptom change; dissociative approaches, which encourages the patient to mentally 'go elsewhere' and leave the pain behind; and resource utilisation, in which the patient uses their internal creativity and imagination.

Management of chronic pain may include all the above, which will be described in some detail later, but also often needs to address co-morbidities such as anxiety, depression or psychosomatic symptomatology. Cognitive behavioural approaches can easily be combined with hypnosis to give more effective outcomes (Jensen et al. 2011).

USING HYPNOSIS TO MANAGE ANXIETY AND DEPRESSION ASSOCIATED WITH CHRONIC PAIN

Teaching patients with chronic pain self-hypnotic techniques can be extremely useful in that it gives them a tool that they can use, not only to help manage their emotions but also to influence their experience of pain.

When someone becomes anxious or depressed there is a pattern in the way they generate their feelings. It may start with an anxious thought or a feeling that then leads to a thought, the thoughts may then generate physiological change, which in turn leads to further thoughts, feelings and behavioural responses. This develops into a vicious spiral of negative feelings and emotions and added to this, the person tends to only notice those things that confirm their emotional state, which further builds the feelings. The patient's focus is then firmly on the anxiety, depression or pain that they are experiencing. Breaking into this pattern in any way possible is the aim of the healthcare professional and the lever to do this will vary from one individual to another.

We get what we focus on, so we need to shift the patient's focus. This could be done through exercise, expressive arts such as music or drawing, painting or colouring, knitting, photography, meditation, social activities or self-hypnosis (and many more). Hypnosis is a very effective way to reduce anxiety and lead the person into a relaxed state (although relaxation is not necessarily a correlate of hypnosis as demonstrated by elite athletes who use hypnotic techniques). Hypnotisability is a genetic trait and follows the normal distribution curve but, as healthcare professionals, we need to work with everyone, not just the top ten percent. Luckily, as with any skill, the ease with which people go into hypnosis improves with practise and one doesn't need any great depth of hypnosis for it to be helpful. Just entering a hypnotic state may help the person to feel more relaxed but the most important part is the giving, and acceptance of, positive suggestions. When someone is new to hypnosis it is useful to use a framework, in the same way as using a recipe when preparing a new dish. Once the person is used to doing self-hypnosis, then closing the eyes, taking a few focusing breaths and setting the intention of going into hypnosis is often sufficient. It is also usually easier to enter the hypnotic state when led by someone but in every case, it is the patient who decides whether or not to follow the suggestions given – the healthcare professional is merely the navigator – the patient is the pilot.

Commonly, the induction of hypnosis may be with an eye roll followed by progressive muscular relaxation, a focus on the breathing or a re-experiencing of an activity in imagination and this initial focusing is followed by suggestions of calmness, control and comfort. It is very easy to induce a hypnotic state; it occurs naturally whenever one finds oneself driving 'on autopilot', or going into a daydream. The important part is what you do with the state once induced. This is why it is important for healthcare practitioners using hypnosis to be competent to work with the conditions they are treating, without hypnosis, before they learn hypnotic techniques as an extra tool in their tool-box. Suggestions are accepted more readily in the hypnotic state and may have an effect long after the hypnosis session has finished. This is useful when post-hypnotic suggestions of calmness and comfort can be used but also means that ill-advised phrases and suggestions can be more harmful than if heard in the normal waking state. Practice is important and it is usual to suggest daily practice of ten to fifteen minutes (or longer) for a few weeks. Scheduling this practice in consultation with the patient can be very helpful and mean they are more likely to do their self-hypnosis on a regular basis. There are many self-hypnosis CD tracks available and some patients find these helpful, especially at first but they do take a variable amount of time and may breed dependency on the tracks used, rather than internalising the skill of self-hypnosis that can be accessed any time the patient feels is appropriate.

It is useful for the patient to develop, in their imagination, a special, calm, peaceful place or safe haven to which they can return when they do their self-hypnosis. This could be a real or an imaginary place, or a mixture of the two. Some people are very visual and have a very clear image of their special place, others only have snatches or an awareness of their place but it is important that they are encouraged to utilise all their senses to really be there and connect with their place. The healthcare practitioner needs to direct the patient to experience whatever they see or hear in their special place, to notice the scents, the temperature, to reach out and touch things there, but above all to really connect with the peace and calmness of the place they have chosen. Nothing goes on in this place that the patient does not control, it is their space that they can go to whenever they need to re-charge their batteries. They could find a keepsake to bring back with them that would instantly remind them of this place and connect them to the calmness. This could be a pebble they imagine holding in their hand, a colour flowing down their body, a phrase they could hear internally or anything else their imagination comes up with. Positive suggestions may be given together with the message that as they practise, it will get easier and quicker to do their self-hypnosis, and that they can bring back the calmness and comfort they are experiencing, as they re-orientate back to the 'here and now'.

If a patient suffers from chronic anxiety the state of relaxation may feel threatening and uncomfortable at first, so a good way to engage with these patients is to ask them to re-experience a physical activity that they have experienced at some time in their life. This could be swimming, cycling horse riding, running, skiing etc. They first of all imagine doing their chosen activity very fast, which matches the high adrenalin state they are used to. All the healthcare professional needs to do is to remind the patient to utilise all their senses to really connect with what they are doing. The patient then begins to slow down their activity at a rate that they are comfortable with until they are floating, resting or doing their activity slowly and easily to a point where they can stop and rest in their special calm place, real or imaginary. They can go and practise this until they are comfortable with it and then maybe experiment with other ways of doing their self-hypnosis.

Patients are sometimes worried about how they will 'wake up' from their self-hypnosis. It is advisable for them to get into the habit of telling themselves how long they are intending to do the self-hypnosis practice for or if they are doing it at bedtime to suggest to themselves that they will drift from hypnosis into a natural sleep and awaken at a certain time, but in any case they would gradually re-orient to their surroundings eventually. If they are sleep deprived, then setting an alarm in case they fall asleep may be useful.

Self-hypnosis is a very useful tool for emotional self-management. If a patient has distressing thoughts, fears, feelings or symptoms that have outlived their usefulness then imagery can be used to get rid of them. If emotions are seen as messages then once the message has been received, we no longer need the emotion. We can focus on feeling an emotion that would be more helpful such as calmness, hope or joy. Some of the many examples of images people have used are of throwing the negative onto a bonfire, down a rubbish chute or into the sea. The negative things may be seen as leaves that you throw into a fast-moving river, or that you attach to a balloon that you send drifting off into the sky. The only limits are the person's imagination. Once having released the negative, the patient needs to connect to the positive and this could be done by finding a pebble or a colour that represents the positive feeling that they need. They could write the positive things somewhere in their special place or in some other way connect themselves to the positive emotion they have decided that they need instead.

Another useful thing for patients to do is to imagine themselves the way they want to be whilst in their special place and connect with it. The goal needs to be realistic, for them to be as healthy as is possible for them, feeling calm and coping better with whatever situation they are in. Having visualised themselves in this way they can step into the image, feeling it and saying something appropriate to themselves. Sometimes their goal is a long way off and it can be useful to suggest that they can see numbered stepping stones (maybe ten) leading to their goal. They can notice which number they are currently standing on and ask internally what they need to do to move one stepping stone nearer to their goal. When they re-orientate they can write down what answer came to them and undertake to do it.

If someone with chronic pain is depressed it may be quite difficult for them to find a happy calm place and the healthcare professional may need to take some time constructing such an imaginary place with the patient. This can always be changed by the patient whenever they wish, as it is their place. Using imagery as described above to discard the negative and connect with positive emotions can be helpful and setting a couple of small goals each day can help the patient feel less overwhelmed. Having a small notebook in which to write down each day where they are on their stepping stones and what goal they are wanting to achieve can be very useful. By writing down the goal and then ticking it off when done, and by writing down the three best things they noticed each day can begin to change their focus of attention to be more positive.

Noticing the positive can be something that can benefit anyone. This could be a flower, a smile, the taste of a good cup of coffee, the feeling of warm water on your back in the shower or anything else. By deliberately noticing these little things we can shift that focus of attention from pain or anxious and depressing thoughts, to outside of ourselves and towards what we are experiencing through our senses of sight, hearing, smell and touch, in the world around us. When someone is anxious, they tend to be focused on possible catastrophes in the future and if depressed tend to ruminate on a negative past, in both cases they do not connect with the present.

Anger may be a factor in chronic pain and this arousal state may exacerbate experienced pain in the same way as stress and anxiety. Anger is rarely constructive but has a destructive effect on the person experiencing it, as opposed to whomever has triggered this response. Having induced hypnosis, the patient is asked to go in their imagination to a rocky place where various rocks are lying around, such as a quarry or a cliff face. They give a nod when they are there and ready to proceed. They are then asked to select a rock and in some way project all the anger that they wish to get rid of into it, maybe marking it in some way so they know what it represents, and to give you a nod when they have done this. They are then asked to look around and see what is available to smash up the rock. There may be a pickaxe, a pneumatic drill, a hammer and chisel, some dynamite or perhaps something else. Once the patient indicates with a nod that they have smashed the rock up, it is important that they then go to a calm peaceful place and remain there until they feel they have really connected to calmness.

HYPNOTIC TECHNIQUES TO RELIEVE PAIN

Hypnotic analgesia is dependent upon suggestion and the induction of hypnosis by itself does not often generate significant pain relief. It is the suggestion inside a hypnotic framework, or at least the expectation of pain relief which leads to reduction of pain. A number of studies have specifically assessed pain relief following a hypnotic induction, or the induction of hypnosis together with specific suggestions (Rainville et al 2008; Zachariae et al. 1998). Dillworth and Jensen (2010) did a literature review and looked at the suggestions given in twenty-five studies where hypnosis was found to be superior to active treatments on a variety of pain-related outcomes. Relaxation alone is not very effective at easing chronic pain (Miller et al. 1991) and various studies looking at forty women suffering from temporomandibular disorders, forty-five patients with fibromyalgia, and twenty-two patients with multiple sclerosis and chronic pain showed that there was decreased pain following hypnotic suggestions for pain relief as compared with simple hypnotic relaxation (Abrahamsen et al. 2009; Jensen et al. 2009; Casetel et al. 2007; Gay et al. 2002).

Jensen and Patterson (2014) reviewed much of the current literature on the use of hypnosis in pain management. They concluded that hypnosis is effective for reducing chronic pain as well as having a number of positive effects beyond pain control. Neurophysiological studies reveal that hypnotic analgesia has clear effects on brain and spinal-cord functioning that differ as a function of the specific hypnotic suggestions made, providing further evidence for the specific effects of hypnosis.

There have been a number of meta-analyses of hypnosis for pain control. Montgomery et al. (2000) examined eighteen studies that revealed a moderate to large hypno-analgesic effect, supporting the efficacy of hypnotic techniques for pain management and Adachi et al. (2014) concluded that hypnosis is efficacious for managing chronic pain.

As well as using imagery in hypnosis to help with the feelings of anxiety and depression often associated with chronic pain, visualisation in hypnosis can also help directly with pain. Derbyshire (2004) demonstrated that hypnotically imagined pain activated the same brain areas as a painful stimulus from a heat probe. This did not happen when the person just imagined the pain out of hypnosis. The implication is, therefore, that if hypnotic suggestion can produce pain, then it can also remove it. This is indeed the case in clinical practice. Although exactly how hypnotic analgesia is produced is not completely understood various studies throw light on possible mechanisms (Fidanza et al. 2017; Derbyshire et al. 2009; Vanhaudenhuyse et al. 2009; Raij et al. 2008; Faymonville et al. 2003; Faymonville et al. 2000) and the beneficial effects last over time (Jensen et al. 2008).

There are numerous studies showing the effectiveness of hypnotic techniques in pain (Tan et al. 2015; Stoelb et al. 2009; Jensen et al. 2009; Abrahamsen et al. 2008; Elkins et al. 2007; Patterson and Jensen 2003). How hypnotic suggestion actually works is unclear but several studies show that the analgesic effect is not reversed by Naloxone in the experimental condition (Moret et al. 1991; Spiegel and Albert 1983; Goldstein and Hilgard 1975).

It can be useful to elicit measures of pain intensity and pain 'bothersomeness' both before, during and after the hypnotic session so that outcomes may be monitored and approaches adjusted accordingly. Often, even if a patient is unable to affect the intensity of the pain, its unpleasantness can be reduced (Rainville et al. 1997).

There are many classic ways of using imagery to reduce pain involving dials and switches but often the most effective way is to engage the patient's unconscious imagery by suggesting that they go down into wherever the pain is and see what image comes to mind as they focus on the discomfort. The healthcare professional then makes the image more 'real' by enquiring about the size, colour, temperature and texture and other aspects. The patient then decides what change would bring some relief. This might be a change in temperature, colour, size or texture.

> As an example, one man with chronic low back pain reported that he needed to sand down the blocks he had visualised and change their colour from red to blue. Over time he did this to his satisfaction and his pain rating dropped considerably. This can be repeated whenever the patient does their self-hypnosis.

Another classic way of using imagery to reduce pain is by imagining warm healing fluid bathing the affected part or by going, in hypnosis, down into a control room in the depths of their mind. Here they can find levers, dials or switches to control inflammation, pain or levels of anxiety or depression. This can be adapted by the patient to their situation and if they are unable to move the dial or lever down, then, continuing their metaphor, they can look to see what is blocking it, or even have a monitor screen upon which they see what they need to deal with before they can reduce their pain.

Simply suggesting that the patient goes and enjoys their special place may be sufficient to reduce pain as the patient dissociates from their painful sensations and really connects with the peaceful place their mind finds for them.

> One woman with terminal ovarian cancer found her last days eased by slipping away in hypnosis to bathe under her warm waterfall whenever she became too uncomfortable.

The time distortion that often occurs in hypnosis may be utilised and suggestions given that the periods of discomfort can become shorter as the periods of comfort in between become so much longer....

If a patient has achieved some degree of comfort in hypnosis then it is important for the healthcare professional to give the post-hypnotic suggestion that the patient can keep this feeling of comfort when they alert and re-orientate themselves. This comfort may also be linked (or anchored) to a phrase, a visual symbol, a sound or even a smell as a conditioned reflex type response. The patient can then use a 'micro-trance' by taking a deep slow breath and bringing their link or anchor to mind in order to connect themselves to a more comfortable state.

> A man with postherpetic neuralgia reduced his discomfort by imagining pouring golden soothing fluid down his nerves and was able to do this whenever he became aware of his neuralgic pain.

For those patients who are highly hypnotisable and able to control their pain in this way it is important that they give themselves the instruction that, if the pain is related to anything that needs their attention, then they will remain aware of it until it is appropriate to reduce it. Analgesic medication also needs to be reduced in a monitored way.

Glove anaesthesia is a well-known hypno-analgesic technique which, as its name implies, follows no anatomical distribution. Suggestions are given to make the patient's hand numb or anaesthetised as a precursor to transferring this numbness to the painful area. There are many ways of doing this either with direct suggestion or using imagery. Imagining in hypnosis the hand becoming cold and numb in icy water or snow, rubbing on a magic numbing cream or pulling on a thick protective glove are commonly used. Metaphors such as being rowed out on a lake and having the patient's hand trail in the water can be used. The patient can choose from these classic approaches or 'do their own thing' but it is worth mentioning to the patient that hypnotic anaesthesia does not mean absence of all sensation but a 'comfortable' numbness can take any sharpness or hurt out of the pain. Once the hand has become numb, the numbness can then be transferred to wherever the pain is situated.

> One woman with chronic neck pain used this technique very successfully to manage her pain that she had had for many years. After three one hour sessions exploring different approaches to managing her nagging cervicalgia and frequent headaches she decided that sitting in her healing pool under her waterfall was soothing but that the easiest (and quickest) way for her was to develop glove anaesthesia (she just used intent and didn't need imagery) and transfer it to the back of her neck. This kept her pain-free for several hours and she then spent a few minutes repeating it as necessary.

Glove anaesthesia is most effective with those who are highly hypnotisable or who have trained themselves in self-hypnosis but many people can obtain a degree of numbness in a surprisingly short time.

UNDERLYING PROBLEMS

As chronic pain has a bio-psycho-social basis, resolving any underlying emotional problems may be a necessary part of management. Often it is found in practice, that once these difficulties have been addressed, the pain no longer poses a problem. Classically these underlying difficulties can be grouped under seven headings: internal conflict; organ language (anatomical metaphors, e.g., back pain may be due to, "I feel I'm being stabbed in the back"); serving an unconscious purpose (secondary gain); past traumatic experience; identification (empathic relationship with someone, who is often deceased); self-punishment; imprint (hetero- or auto- suggestion accepted virtually unchallenged at a time of great stress or when in shock). These can all be explored in hypnosis and resolved in ways appropriate for the patient and the situation. If the health professional is intending to use hypnosis in this way, more training and experience is required, not only in hypnosis but more importantly in counselling and psychology.

> One woman complaining of Fibromyalgia had suppressed feelings of anger and loss surrounding her divorce of her alcoholic husband and estrangement from her daughter. Once she had worked through her feelings about these past events over a couple of sessions, her fibromyalgia no longer troubled her and she was still well when seen five years later.
> A thirty seven year old man presented with chronic lower back pain. When seen he reported that he had hurt his back, shifting furniture, five years previously and suffered with back pain since. He rated its intensity as varying between 4 and 9 on a ten-point scale. Around the time he started with back pain he discovered that his business partner was embezzling money from the company and he was struggling to keep the company solvent. In hypnosis he described his pain as feeling as if he was being stabbed in the back. After working through his feelings of loss and anger at what had happened his back was greatly improved and he continued to use imagery when he did self-hypnosis to remain virtually pain-free. As his pain receded, he undertook more exercise and this would also have contributed to his good outcome.
> A sixty year old woman presented with postherptic neuralgia that she had had for twelve years. She described the pain as being as if someone was rubbing salt into an open wound in her side. On using hypnosis to explore any underlying factor contributing to her pain she described how the doctor had told her that she would always have neuralgia pain and that there was no cure. This may not have been the historic truth but it is what

she interpreted from what she heard. The language we use is not simply a description of our reality – it actively constructs it. In hypnosis the patient was able to observe what had happened and realise that what she heard was not what had been intended and was, in any case, merely the doctor's opinion. She was then able to use imagery very successfully to feel more comfortable.

A man of thirty four had been involved in a serious road traffic accident four years previously and although no physical cause had been found, he suffered from constant headaches. On exploring what had happened he recalled that he had been lying in the wreckage of his car waiting for the firemen to release him and had had the thought that he must still be alive because his head hurt. At some level his mind had linked being alive with headache so logically he needed the headaches to be sure he was alive! Once he had allowed that younger part of him that had had the accident to really know that he had come through it and was okay he didn't need the headaches any more. He was able to stop his analgesic medication.

CONCLUSION

Hypnosis can be a useful tool in the management of chronic pain as well as any associated emotional distress.

Hypnosis may be used informally by engaging the patient's imagination and giving suggestion through conversational means but usually when working with patients with chronic pain it is used in a sessional context. Building rapport with the patient and dispelling any misconceptions the patient may have regarding hypnosis is necessary before self-hypnosis and uses of imagery can be taught. Although inducing the hypnotic state may be relatively simple, it is important to know how to utilise it effectively using suggestion and imagery. An understanding of the patient's clinical condition and some counselling or psychological training are essential. There is no statutory regulation of hypnosis in the UK and many organisations offer hypnosis training of varying standards. There is only one not for profit organisation in England that is run solely by and for healthcare professionals. BSCAH (The British Society of Clinical & Academic

Hypnosis) runs training courses for qualified healthcare professionals and also a university Advanced Diploma with the City of Birmingham University. Details of trainings can be found at www.bscah.com. For the safety of patients and practitioners alike BSCAH only supports the use of hypnosis to treat conditions that the healthcare professional is competent to treat within their field of expertise without hypnosis.

Although there is an increasing body of evidence for the use of hypnosis in many clinical contexts, there is great need for further good quality studies to support its use in cancer pain and other chronic pain conditions. The main difficulty is obtaining funding as hypnosis is not regarded as a mainstream approach and it is very difficult to double blind delivery of a therapeutic intervention that is as tailored to the individual as hypnosis is. Random controlled trials were developed to access the efficacy of medications where it is much easier to reduce variables to a minimum. Also, the motivation is very different for those taking part in a laboratory experiment compared to that within the clinical context and fortunately within the clinical field the majority of patients can benefit to some extent, some quite spectacularly.

Those who use hypnotic techniques within their practice are well aware of how effective and useful it can be and how it often speeds up therapeutic interventions. This chapter will hopefully have shown some of the increasing evidence for its use in chronic pain and by describing simply some of the easier hypnotic interventions, encourage more healthcare professionals to seek training in this useful and versatile tool. Within the anaesthetic field it has certainly been shown to be cost-effective (Lang and Rosen 2002) and once self-hypnosis has been taught to a patient, they have a tool that can help with self-management for life.

REFERENCES

Abrahamsen R, L Baad-Hansen and P Svensson. 2008. "Hypnosis in the management of persistent idiopathic orofacial pain – clinical and psychosocial findings." *Pain,* 136, no1-2. (May): 44–52.

Abrahamsen R, R Zachariae and P Svensson. 2009. "Effect of hypnosis on oral function and psychological factors in temporomandibular disorders patients." *Journal of Oral Rehabilitation*. 36, no 8. (August): 556-7.

Adachi T, H Fujino, A Nakae, T Mashimo and J Sasaki. 2014. "A meta-analysis of hypnosis for chronic pain problems: a comparison between hypnosis, standard care, and other psychological interventions." *International Journal of Clinical and Experimental Hypnosis*, 62 no 1: 1-28.

Bair M, R Robinson, W Katon, and K Kroenke. 2003. "Depression and Pain Comorbidity: A Literature Review." *Archives of Internal Medicine American Medical Association*. 163, no 20. (November): 2433-2445.

Brann L. 2012 "Explanation of Hypnosis: The Working Model" in *The Handbook of Contemporary Clinical Hypnosis* edited by L Brann, J Owens and A Williamson. 97-105. Chichester, W Sussex: Wiley-Blackwell.

Bushnell C, M Ceko and L Low. 2013. "Cognitive and emotional control of pain and its disruption in chronic pain." *Nature Reviews Neuroscience* 14, no 7 (July): 502–511.

Castel A, M Perez, J Sala, A Padrol and M Rull. 2007. "Effect of hypnotic suggestion on fibromyalgic pain: Comparison between hypnosis and relaxation." *European Journal of Pain*. 11, no 4. (May): 463–468.

Chaput J. 2014. "Sleep patterns, diet quality and energy balance." *Physiology & Behaviour* 134. (July): 86-91. https://doi: 10.1016/j.physbeh.2013.09.006.

Derbyshire S, M Whalley, V Stenger and D Oakley. 2004. "Cerebral activation during hypnotically induced and imagined pain." *NeuroImage*, 23, no 1. (September): 392-401.

Derbyshire S, M Whalley, and D Oakley. 2009. "The nature of fibromyalgia pain and the role of hypnosis and suggestion in its alleviation: an fMRI study." *European Journal of Pain*, 13, no 5. (May): 542-50.

Dillworth T and M Jensen. 2010. "The Role of Suggestions in Hypnosis for Chronic Pain: A Review of the Literature." *The open pain journal* 3, no 1; 39-51.

Elkins G, M Jensen and D Patterson. 2007. "Hypnotherapy for the Management of Chronic Pain." *International Journal of Clinical and Experimental Hypnosis*, 55, no 3. (July): 275–287.

Fayaz A, P Croft, R Langford, L Donaldson and G Jones. 2016. "Prevalence of chronic pain in the UK: a systematic review and meta-analysis of population studies." *BMJ Open* 6, no (6) e010364. (June) https://doi:10.1136/bmjopen-2015-010364.

Faymonville M E, S Laureys, C Degueldre, G Fiore, A Luxen, G Franck, M Lamy and P Maquet. 2000. "Neural mechanisms of antinociceptive effects of hypnosis." *Anesthesiology*, 92, no 5. (May) 1257-1267.

Faymonville M E, L Roediger, G Fiore, C Delgueldre, C Phillips, M Lamy, A Luxen, P Maquet and S Laureys. 2003. "Increased cerebral functional connectivity underlying the antinociceptive effects of hypnosis." *Brain Research. Cognitive Brain Research,* 17, no 2. (July): 255-262.

Fidanza F, M Varanini, A Ciaramella, G Carli and E Santarcangelo. 2017. "Pain modulation as a function of hypnotizability: Diffuse noxious inhibitory control induced by cold pressor test vs explicit suggestions of analgesia." *Physiology & Behavior,* 171. (February): 135-141.

Fishbain D, R Cutler, H Rosomoff, R S Rosomoff. 1997. "Chronic Pain-Associated Depression: Antecedent or Consequence of Chronic Pain? A Review" *The Clinical Journal of Pain,* 13, no 2 (June): 116-137.

Gay M-C, P Philippot and O Lumine. 2002. "Differential effectiveness of psychological interventions for reducing osteoarthritis pain: a comparison of Erickson hypnosis and Jacobson relaxation." *European Journal of Pain*, 6: 1-16.

Goldstein A and E Hilgard. 1975. "Failure of opiate antagonist Naloxone to modify hypnotic analgesia." *Proceedings of the National Academy of Sciences. USA*, 6: 2041-2043.

Jensen M, J Barber, M Hanley, J Engel, J Romano, D Cardenas, G Kraft, A Hoffman A and D Patterson. 2008. "Long-term outcome of hypnotic-analgesia treatment for chronic pain in persons with disabilities." *International Journal of Clinical and Experimental Hypnosis,* 56, no 2:156-69.

Jensen M, J Barber, J Romano, I Molton, K Raichle, T Osborne, J Engel, B Stoelb, G Kraft, and D Patterson. 2009. "A comparison of self-hypnosis versus progressive muscle relaxation in patients with multiple sclerosis and chronic pain." *The International Journal of Clinical and Experimental Hypnosis.* 57, no 2. (April): 198-221.

Jensen M, J Barber, J Romano, M Hanley, K Raichle, I Molton, J Engel, T Osborne, B Stoelb, D Cardenas and D Patterson. 2009. "Effects of self-hypnosis training and EMG biofeedback relaxation training on chronic pain in persons with spinal-cord injury." *The International Journal of Clinical and Experimental Hypnosis,* 57, no 3. (July): 239-68.

Jensen M, D Ehde, K Gertz, B Stoelb, T Dillworth, A Hirsh, I Molton, and G Kraft. 2011. "Effects of self-hypnosis training and cognitive restructuring on daily pain intensity and catastrophizing in individuals with multiple sclerosis and chronic pain." *The International Journal of Clinical and Experimental Hypnosis*, 59, no 1. (January): 45-63.

Jensen M and D Patterson. 2014. "Hypnotic approaches for chronic pain management: clinical implications of recent research findings." *American Psychologist,* 69 no 2: 167-177.

Kihlstrom J. 1985. "Hypnosis." *Annual Review of Psychology.* 36, (February): 385-418.

Kosslyn S, W Thompson, M Constantin-Ferrando, N Alpert and D Spiegel. 2000. "Hypnotic visual illusion alters colour processing in the brain." *American Journal of Psychiatry.* 157, no 8. (August): 1279-84.

Lang E and M Rosen. 2002. "Cost analysis of adjunct hypnosis with sedation during outpatient interventional radiologic procedures." *Radiology*, 222, no 2: 375-82.

Lebon J, M. Rongiéres, C. Apredoaei, S. Declaux, and P. Mansat. 2017. "Physical therapy under hypnosis for the treatment of patients with type 1 complex regional pain syndrome of the hand and wrist: Retrospective study of 20 cases." *Hand Surgery Rehabilitation*, 36 no 3. (June):215-221.

Miller M, A Barabasz and M Barabasz. 1991. "Effects of active alert and relaxation hypnotic inductions on cold pressor pain." *Journal of Abnormal Psychology*, 100, no 2: 223-226.

Montgomery G, K DuHamel, and W Redd. 2000. "A meta-analysis of hypnotically induced analgesia: how effective is hypnosis?" *International Journal of Clinical and Experimental Hypnosis,* 48 no 2. (April): 138-53.

Moret V, A Forster, M Laverrière, H Lambert, R Gaillard, P Bourgeois, A Haynal, M Gemperle and E Buchser. 1991. "Mechanism of analgesia induced by hypnosis and acupuncture: is there a difference?" *Pain,* 45, no 2 (May):135-40.

Moseley G. 2003. "A pain neuromatrix approach to patients with chronic pain." *Manual Therapy* 8. no 3 (August):130-40.

Patterson D and M Jensen. 2003. "Hypnosis and clinical pain." *Psychological Bulletin,* 129, no 4. (July): 495-521.

Petrie K, J Müller, F Schirmbeck, L Donkin, E Broadbent, C Ellis, G Gamble and W Rief. 2007. "Effect of providing information about normal test results on patients' reassurance: randomised controlled trial." *British Medical Journal.* 17, (February) 334(7589): 352.

Pintar J and S Lynn. 2008. *"Hypnosis: A Brief History."* (September) Wiley-Blackwell.

Raij T, J Numminen, S Narvarnen, J Hiltunen and R Hari. (2005). "Brain correlates of subjective reality of physically and psychologically induced pain." *Proceedings of the National Academy of Sciences of the United States of America,* 102, no 6. (February): 2147-2151.

Rainville P, G Duncan, D Price, B Carrier and M Bushnell. 1997. "Pain affect encoded in the human anterior cingulate but not somatosensory cortex." *Science,* 277: 988-71.

Rainville Pierre. 2008. "Hypnosis and the analgesic effect of suggestions." *Pain,* 134, no 1-2 (February): 1-2.

Richter M, J Eck, T Straube, W Miltner and T Weiss. 2010. "Do words hurt? Brain activation during the processing of pain-related words." *Pain,* 148, no 2. (February):198-205.

Spiegel D and L Albert. 1983. "Naloxone fails to reverse hypnotic alleviation of chronic pain." *Psychopharmacology* (Berl), 81, no 2:140-3.

Stoelb B, I Molton, M Jensen and D Patterson. 2009. "The efficacy of hypnotic analgesia in adults: a review of the literature." *Contemporary Hypnosis*, 26 no 1. (March): 24-39.

Tan G, D Rintala, M Jensen, T Fukui, D Smith and W Williams. 2015. "A randomized controlled trial of hypnosis compared with biofeedback for adults with chronic low back pain." *European Journal of Pain*, 19, no 2. (February): 271-80.

Vanhaudenhuyse A, M Boly, E Balteau, C Schnakers, G Moonen, A Luxen, M Lamy, C Degueldre, J Brichant, P Maquet, S Laureys and M E Faymonville. 2009. "Pain and non-pain processing during hypnosis: A thalium-YAG event-related fMRI study." *NeuroImage*, 47, no 3. (September): 1047-1054.

Zachariae R, O Andersen, P Bjerring and M Jorgensen. 1998. "Effects of an opioid antagonist on pain intensity and withdrawal reflexes during induction of hypnotic analgesia in high- and low-hypnotizable volunteers." *European Journal of Pain*. 2, no 1. (April): 25-34.

BIOGRAPHICAL SKETCH

Dr Ann Williamson studied at Bristol University, obtaining her MB ChB in 1972. She was a General Practitioner for thirty two years at Pennine Medical Centre, Mossley, Lancashire from 1974 and has used hypnosis since the late 1980s to help her patients deal with stress and anxiety and to help them facilitate change in how they live their lives. She is an Accredited member of the British Society of Clinical & Academic Hypnosis (BSCAH), a certified NLP Master Practitioner and has had training in brief solution oriented therapy and other approaches. She has been involved for many years with (BSCAH) teaching Health Professionals how to use hypnotic techniques both for themselves and within their own field of clinical expertise. She runs stress management, personal development and brief psychological interventions workshops on request, as well as seeing private clients for therapy. She has also lectured at Manchester, Chester and Salford Universities as well as in Canada and Europe. She has written three books:

on stress management, smoking cessation and on brief psychological interventions in clinical practice. She is also co-editor of A Handbook of Contemporary Hypnosis published by Wiley in 2011 and has contributed to several other books and journals. She is also a Reiki Master Trainer and has an interest in creativity and exploring one's emotions through the arts.

For more details please visit www.annwilliamson.co.uk

- *Smoke free – no buts*, Co-author, (1998) Crown House Publishing Ltd. ISBN: 1-899836-20-9.
- *Still – in the Storm*, (1999) Crown House Publishing Ltd. ISBN: 189983641-1.
- Reprinted 2000, 2004; translated into Russian, Chinese and Spanish.
- Named contributor to *Hypnosis, Dissociation and Survivors of Child Abuse* by Marcia Degun-Mather, (2006) Wiley. ISBN: 0-470-01945-X.
- *Brief Psychological Interventions in Practice*, (2008) Wiley, ISBN: 978-0-470-51306-4.
- *The Handbook of Contemporary Clinical Hypnosis: Theory and Practice*, L Brann, J Owens & A Williamson (2011) Wiley-Blackwell, Chichester, ISBN 978-0-470-68367-5.
- Named contributor to *Hypnotherapy: A Handbook* by Michael Heap (2012) Open University Press, ISBN: 0335244459.
- Brief Psychological and Hypnotic Interventions in Chronic Pain Management. (2016) *J Contemp Psychother* 46 (3):179-186. Springer.
- What is hypnosis and how might it work? (2019) *Palliative Care: Research and Treatment* https://doi.org/10.1177/1178224219826581.

In: Chronic Pain
Editor: Stefan Friedman

ISBN: 978-1-53616-296-7
© 2019 Nova Science Publishers, Inc.

Chapter 2

THE JOURNEY TO COPING: A GROUNDED THEORY OF PAIN COPING AMONGST MALTESE CHRONIC PAIN SUFFERERS

Pamela Portelli[1],* and Clare Eldred[2]
[1]Psychology Department, University of Malta, Gozo, Malta
[2]Department of Social Sciences, City University, London, UK

ABSTRACT

This chapter comprises a study exploring pain coping mechanisms amongst Maltese chronic pain patients. Semi-structured interviews were conducted with 21 participants. Findings derived from a grounded theory methodology revealed that Maltese often display a seeming reluctance to rely on pharmacological therapies, relying on a number of self-taught/sought strategies. The journey to coping is not an easy one, with some participants engaging in relentless struggles to eliminate pain. The inability to achieve control often leads to a sense of disconnectedness from the external world. Sometimes, death by suicide is perceived as the only solution, albeit an unacceptable one. Although religion may be a protective

---

* Corresponding Author's E-mail: pamela.portelli.1@city.ac.uk.

factor against suicide, it also seemed a major impediment because participants perceived suicide as sinful in the eyes of God. On the other hand, effective self-preservation strategies can foster a sense of acceptance. The importance of taking into account the religious and cultural dimension in the pain experience was identified.

Keywords: adaptation, coping, enduring, chronic illness and disease, chronic pain

INTRODUCTION

Pain is an inevitable and unavoidable universal human experience. Although unpleasant, it is of vital importance for the body in reducing the impact of potential physical damage (Sarafino & Smith 2014). Pain becomes problematic when it is chronic and enduring and when it impairs the quality of life of the individual. Bio-psychosocial approaches shed light on the complexity of chronic pain, emphasizing the interdependence of biological, psychological and social factors in pain perception. Understanding somatic manifestations of pain requires a consideration of multidimensional and contextual circumstances.

Despite advances in medical treatment, unrelieved pain remains a challenge. Given the widespread implications of chronic pain, an ideal treatment would encompass a multi-disciplinary approach. Unfortunately, specialization and expansion of services is not always possible, the Maltese islands being a case in point, where services revolve mainly round conventional medical treatments (Azzopardi et al. 2012). There are two pain clinics on the Maltese islands, one situated at Mater Dei Hospital and one at Gozo General Hospital. The specialized pain clinics at the local hospitals are run on an out-patients basis by 5 pain management consultants, each one having their own nurse. Services revolve mainly round the administration of medication, referral to acupuncture, transcutaneous electrical nerve stimulation and physiotherapy. No psychological services are currently available at the pain clinics.

Qualitative research has explored how individuals cope with pain. A qualitative study revealed that coping comprises a long-term process of building self-determination to live a life in accordance with one's values (Hamilton 2010). Participants in the latter study suffered from endometriosis and conclusively, results are only true for the aforementioned population. Another study on older adults experiencing leg ulceration by (Taverner et al. 2014) reveals that adaptation to chronic pain comprises a phase-like trajectory comprising a host of psychosocial repercussions including depression, reduced quality of life and desire for amputation.

According to Engel's bio-psychosocial model (1977) cultural factors play a significant role in pain behaviours. Conclusively, the phenomenon of pain cannot be studied in isolation without taking into account the surrounding context. What may be the norm in one context, could perhaps be seen as totally inappropriate in another cultural setting. Pain coping amongst the Maltese is poorly understood, mainly because no input from the Maltese perspective has been incorporated into existing pain coping theories. Although diverse psychological models and theories shed light on the complexity of pain coping, they all have their limitations. Engel's (1977) bio-psychosocial model falls short of providing a comprehensive explanation of pain coping because it ignores the spiritual and subjective nature of pain and the way individuals attempt to make meaning of life with pain. On the other hand, although the Bio-psychosocial-spiritual Model of Health (Hiatt 1986) incorporates a spiritual domain, it does not address the theme of chronic pain (Hamilton 2010). Despite universal coping strategies, individuals often adopt unique ways of coping, based on culturally accepted values and norms (Lam & Zane, 2004). Illness representations are influenced by the person's perceptions, attitudes, experiences and beliefs which are in turn affected by socio-cultural factors including services available within a given community, access to health care, socio-economic status and significant others (Evans & Kazarain 1989). Cultural influences in pain behaviour and their consequences have been neglected, particularly among a Maltese population.

The Maltese culture is a rich one, comprising beliefs and practices resulting from the process of adaptation of different societies that came in contact with the Maltese islands throughout history. The Maltese tongue is influenced by the succession of diverse northern and southern rulers, making Maltese culture unique. Following the shipwreck of St. Paul in 60AD, Malta remains a very devout Roman Catholic nation. According to recent data, 95% of the Maltese population is Roman Catholic, with the remaining 5% being followers of other religious affiliations (Gouder 2010). These historic processes have resulted in a culture comprising an ethnic admixture that defines Maltese identity. Given cultural disparities in pain behaviours, the ethnic admixture defining Maltese identity and the profound impact of religion on the Maltese culture, this study will therefore explore pain coping amongst this population. Although some similarities with other populations are to be expected, coping preferences unique to the Maltese population alongside an explanatory coping process model are discussed.

METHODOLOGY

Intensive semi-structured interviews were employed to provide a rich account of participants' lived experiences (Charmaz 2000). Open-ended interview questions serve as guidelines to explore the topic at hand. This facilitates open interactional space for ideas and issues to arise (Charmaz 2000). Most pain coping research employs quantitative methodologies to score and code people's replies (Been et al. 2016), thereby falling short of providing an in-depth understanding of the complex bio-psychosocial phenomena behind people's behaviours and perceptions. Quantitative approaches adopt observable measures to describe hypothetical and unobservable constructs that are difficult to quantify (Hewstone et al. 1997), pain coping being a case in point. A major criticism of these methods is their emphasis on theory verification, hypothetic-deductive approach and relentless search for objective reality. These are major obstacles to thinking and discovery (Rennie et al. 1988). Qualitative methodologies enable researchers to go beyond theory verification by creating new theories in areas where knowledge is lacking or sparse (Rennie et al. 1988).

This research aims to understand the meaning behind human behaviour in the field of chronic pain, an area which may be difficult to access using traditional research methods. Existing theories that are often applied to conceptualize strategies in relation to pain coping include Lazarus & Folkman's (1984) model of stress. Nevertheless, they fail to provide an in-depth exploration of meaningful constructs that play a role in pain coping and the uptake of psychological services. Pain coping is complicated by factors such as gender, socio-cultural factors, severity of the problem and the socioeconomic circumstances of the individual. This research aimed to integrate all these constructs into a coherent whole. Grounded theory (Charmaz 2000) was identified as the best methodology to use. It is well equipped to investigate socially-related phenomena. This bottom-up approach to research originally developed by Glaser & Strauss (1968) is based on an inductive approach to data analysis and aims to achieve higher levels of understanding via the development of new theories emerging from the data.

Over time, related yet divergent disciplinary traditions of the methodology have emerged. Charmaz's (2000) constructivist approach asserts that the researcher and participants play an active role in constructing research. Research is constructed rather than discovered (Charmaz 2000). Conclusively, researchers' reflexivity plays a crucial role in the process of data analysis. Stereotypical norms and expectations influence differences in pain expression and behaviour (Keogh et al. 2004). Moreover, although pain is subjective, individuals of similar cultural backgrounds tend to display similar pain responses (Davidhizar & Giger 2004). Traditional pain coping research often relies on methods that take responses out of context and ignore the ways meanings are constructed in ordinary talk (Langdridge & Taylor 2007). Pain coping is formed within a social context and is therefore the result of social processes. An investigation of the lived experience of pain incorporates the social and interpretative element. Different researchers may come up with different interpretations of participants' experiences. For the reasons outlined above, it was felt that Charmaz's constructivist approach to grounded theory was the best method to use.

Participants

11 males and 10 females participated in this study. The average age was 52 years. All participants were Maltese. Inclusion criteria were being over 18 years, have been suffering from a pain condition lasting more than 3 months (to fit the IASP diagnostic criteria), be of Maltese nationality and currently receiving services from the local pain clinic. Interview duration lasted between 28-58 minutes. Table 1 provides illustrates type of chronic pain experienced by participants and gender.

Table 1. Pain condition by gender

Pain condition	Males	Females
Fibromyalgia	0	5
Degenerative Disc Disease	1	1
Backpain	3	4
Sciatic nerve inflammation	1	0
Neurofibromatosis/syringomyelia	1	0
Unexplained chronic headache	1	0
Abdominal pain	1	1
Arthritis	2	2
Complex Regional Pain Syndrome	1	0
Scoliosis	0	1

Note: (some participants suffered from more than one pain condition)

Interview Guide

Demographics and other information related to presenting problem were collected prior to the interview. Following a pilot interview, an interview guide using open-ended neutral questions was finalized. Sample interview questions included:

> Can you describe your pain? What kind of treatments you have you sought so far and to what extent have they been helpful? What is it like to live with pain on a day to day basis and how is it affecting you? What do you do to cope?

Procedure and Recruitment

Details of the study and contact details of the research were placed on posters in the local pain clinic. Potential participants who expressed an interest in the study contacted the researcher. They were then assessed for inclusion criteria. A brief description of the aims, eligibility criteria, method of data collection, duration and contact details were provided. This process resulted in the recruitment of 21 participants. Participants were requested to read and sign a consent sheet explaining that participation was voluntary and that they could withdraw at any stage. The anticipated duration of the interview was also highlighted. They could refrain from answering a particular question if they felt uncomfortable doing so. Only questions related to the topic at hand were asked. The recruitment process and data collection lasted four months. Interviews were done by a doctoral psychology student who was trained in research methods. Data analysis was done in collaboration with a university academic with a doctoral degree in psychology. Interviews were conducted at the local hospital pain clinic while participants were waiting to be seen by the pain management consultant. This process helped eliminate some barriers to data collection such as transport problems and problems finding a venue for the interview. Interviews lasted between thirty minutes to an hour fifteen minutes. One was terminated due to the participant being in pain. Interviews were audio-recorded. No remuneration was provided.

Ethical Issues

Ethical approval was obtained from City University London Ethics Committee and the University Research Ethics Committee (UREC) of the University of Malta. Participants were treated according to the British Psychological Society's ethics code (2009). Confidentiality was ensured. Participants were requested to read and sign a consent sheet with information about the aims of the study and what participation entailed. Consent and information sheets were available in both English and Maltese. It was explained that participation was voluntary and that they could withdraw at any stage without suffering adverse consequences. In order to safeguard both researcher and participants, interviews were done throughout the day when the hospital Crisis Team was still operating. Data was locked in a safe place. There was no need for follow-up interviews. Contact details for additional support were provided.

The Process of Data Collection and Theory Building

Following the identification of the topic, the second step in grounded theory methodology involves the formulation of open-ended and neutral questions. Interview questions were based on findings from successive narratives to build a theory grounded in data. Themes raised by participants were followed up in subsequent interviews with new participants, thereby allowing data collection and interpretation to proceed in parallel. This allowed emergent themes to be explored in more detail in successive interviews. The first two interviews were held on the same day, yielding very rich data. Although the same set of questions were used here, the researcher allowed for a degree of flexibility and used gentle probing to elicit further information about significant points raised by participants. It also allowed for a slight modification of questions asked in the interviews conducted after them. For instance, the psychological effects pain was having on the participants' lives became very evident. As a result, a question on perceptions of the role of psychological factors in pain coping was explored in successive narratives. The theme of spiritual coping was also strongly felt and delved into in other interviews.

In the present study, theoretical sampling was used to expand the categories developed during the process of data collection. This was done by seeking out interviews with a wide range of participants who might be expected to give different accounts from those already collected (e.g., those who had a clear diagnosis and with unexplained pain, different treatment trajectories, participants of different gender, educational background and gender) and through more focused questioning around the concepts as they emerged. Variation facilitates in-depth exploration of dimensions and relations as well as theoretical sampling and constant comparative analysis (Oktay 2012). Memos were used as part of the analytic process of the development of categories and their inter-relationships.

Keeping in line with the principles of theoretical sampling, constant comparative analysis was used whereby data was collected over a four-month period. This iterative process allows theory building to evolve (Oktay 2012). Data was transcribed and analysed after each interview. Additional data was gathered at different points to ensure further development and concept verification. No predetermined sample size was identified since this can interfere with the process of theory building, resulting in the omission of potentially rich and important information (Oktay 2012). Moreover, the researcher cannot know in advance when the saturation point will be reached. Data collection continued until the researcher felt that no new themes were emerging in the last few interviews conducted. Samples comprising 20 participants, or more are considered reasonable for grounded theory (Creswell 1998). For the latter reasons, data saturation was considered to have been achieved following interview 21. This was also due to the fact that the research question was quite focused and specific.

In line with recommendations for increasing validity of responses in qualitative research (Brink 1993), it was ensured that participants had a clear understanding of the nature of the study. Written records were also reviewed and confirmed with participants for completeness and accuracy of data. The latter was done by scheduling an appointment with participants at a time that was convenient them and researcher.

Procedures for Data Analysis

Interview data was translated, transcribed verbatim and typed up with wide margins for note-taking during the coding process. This included facial expressions, tone of voice and body language conveying information pertinent to the participants' intended meaning. Data analysis in grounded theory entails coming up with an initial research question(s) for data collection, followed by an analysis of the unstructured material, further data collected and analysis as required, the setting up of theoretical categories towards more ordered analytical concepts and theory establishment. Memos taken were used throughout to ensure theoretical sensitivity and that interviews were fresh in the researcher's mind. Memos allowed the researcher to record initial impressions on the data. For instance, at one point one participant started talking about the death of her son. She said the fibromyalgia appeared a few months after that. The author started wondering whether the physical pain could also be a manifestation of emotional pain and the loss she had endured. The stages for data analysis are illustrated below.

Open Coding

Interviews were re-read several times to allow for increased familiarity with data. No coding scheme was set up prior to the process of data collection to avoid forcing data into pre-existing categories (Oktay 2012). Emerging key words, responses, thoughts and associations were noted. Line-by-line initial coding with gerunds was used as a heuristic device to bring the researcher closer to the data, allow interaction and further fragmentation. Themes and categories were recorded and coded into smaller chunks according to their meaning and relevance to the study (Strauss & Corbin, 1990).

Focused Coding

This process entailed using the most significant and frequent earlier identified codes to sift through and analyse large amounts of data. This stage was an emergent process since unexpected ideas were uncovered. Information was verified alongside the original transcripts to ensure categories were an accurate reflection of participants' replies and to facilitate higher level analysis. Data was reassembled by drawing attention to relationships and shared meanings. Memos and categories were hand-written on individual cards and scattered on a large table. This process facilitated the process of linking concepts in a meaningful manner. For instance, following a deeper analysis of data, the initial sub-category'

Restoring Homeostasis' was changed to *'Adapting to a Modified me'*. Thus, rather than finding the lost self, it became evident that participants who had accepted their pain and were coping better had managed to *'let go'* of what was and found new ways of living in a body with pain.

Selective Coding

This entails integrating and identifying core categories to form an overarching theory. Constant comparative method was used where data coding was performed until a strong theoretical understanding emerged (Boeiji 2002).

Reflexivity

Reflexivity is an ongoing evaluative process in data collection (Guillemin & Gillam 2004). It requires a reflection on personal perspectives and biases that may influence knowledge construction.

The phenomenon of chronic pain is not novel to a health psychologist. As a result, it is difficult to totally distance oneself from what one already knows about the subject matter. Nonetheless, as Dey (1999) rightly points out, *'prior conceptions need not become preconceptions*. Efforts were made to reduce the contamination of emergent data. A reflective diary was kept during the process of data collection. Initial questions asked were general, aiming to elicit information about the kind and type of pain experienced as well as its duration. As more specific factors related to coping started to emerge, questions became more focused on the topic at hand as narrated by the participants. The researcher tried to remain open to what was happening in the interview by listening to participants' narratives and concerns. As a health psychology researcher, the author recalls feeling frustrated upon finding out about the lack of psychological input in local pain clinics. Thus, to the question *'What is the role of psychological factors in the experience of pain?'*, caution was exercised in relation to the paradox she could have shared with participants, particularly those who did not share similar views. An effort was made to maintain a neutral stance without impinging personal views both during data collection. A conscious effort was also made to avoid providing health-related advice as this could have contaminated the data by making participants alter their account to conform to the researcher's expectations rather than being true to their own experiences and feelings. It posed the risk of promoting oneself as a superior source of health knowledge and expertise, thereby creating a power imbalance between participants and the researcher.

Since this study recruited Maltese participants, interviews had to be translated from the native language to English. A way of increasing research validity in translation involves developing culturally competent knowledge (Meleis 1996) or a good understanding of the language variations adopted by the target population. Familiarity with the culture of participants is also crucial (Vuilliamy 1990). Since the researcher was Maltese and bilingual, the translation process was facilitated. A pilot interview ensured a smoother translation process (Birbili 2000). Data from the latter was not included since the participant had not been suffering for chronic pain long enough to meet inclusion criteria. An English language teacher was also consulted since the latter reduces translation bias (Birbili 2000) and disagreements were resolved by mutual agreement.

The researcher was aware that the kind of questions asked and how they were asked could shape participants' replies. For instance, asking too many questions and providing unintentional verbal signals about how the interview was progressing could result in her dominating the interview process. Some precautions were taken to reduce direction of content. Initial questions were broad and general, with occasional prompts and minimum interference from behalf of the researcher. The researcher reflected back on participants' narratives in order to check for understanding, gain further insight and clarify meanings.

RESULTS

This section presents findings derived from the adoption of a bottom-up grounded theory methodology. Three main themes identified were i) developing strategies for self-preservation and re-attaining wellness ii) acquiescing to pain as a stronger force and iii) accepting pain into sense of self. These will be presented with discussion of their associated sub-themes'. Pseudonyms have been used throughout.

Developing Strategies for Self-Preservation and Re-Attaining Wellness

Escalating pain propels individuals to seek pain alleviation, mostly via pharmacological treatments. When the latter fail, individuals often end up self-medicating. Different coping strategies were further divided into the following eight subthemes.

Thought Regulation
This included distraction, positive imagery, focusing on the here and now and distraction as evident in the excerpts below:

> 'Whenever I notice that I am starting to feel stressed and to think negatively....I imagine I am by the sea...I imagine I am near the mountains (smiles)...I imagine where I would like to be in the present moment...that helps me see the positive side of things'. (Rose)
> 'I feel so engrossed in the conversation right now that I don't feel any pain!' (Brian)

Reframing was another coping strategy:

> 'It is true I am in pain...but...it is not a serious and life-threatening illness...it is not like cancer, for instance.'(Brian)

Routine and Behaviour Change
These include keeping well-informed, having a routine, avoiding over-exertion, relaxation, meditation, tapping, having a hot shower, yoga and

engaging in self-care. For instance, one participant modified her eating habits:

> 'I had to change my diet...I went to see a nutritionist...she told me to avoid acidic foods...I did feel a bit better after modifying my diet.'(Maria)

On the other hand, unhealthy coping strategies included binging, over-exertion and smoking.

Physical Therapy
This comprised stretching exercises, physiotherapy, walking and swimming.

> 'I obviously do my daily exercises...being a physiotherapist means I know what needs to be done.' (Mary Doris)

Stimulation Therapies
These included transcutaneous electrical nerve stimulation and acupuncture for pain relief.

Self-Sought and Self-Taught Symptom Management
Some participants engaged in self-experimentation for pain relief.

> 'I even tried a gel which is usually used on horses...and believe it or not...it is the one which was the most effective.'(Joe)

Keeping up to Date and Assimilating Knowledge
The internet was used to ensure one was well-informed about one's condition and up-to-date with the most innovative treatments. Sometimes, it was used as a self-diagnostic tool or to confirm a given diagnosis. A prevalent belief was that 'the internet has revolutionized the world' and that some problems could easily be prevented if one is well informed.

Reaching out to a Higher Power

Females were more likely to express reliance on religious coping. Religion seems to serve diverse purposes including a source of comfort during episodes of unbearable pain. Praying helped participants find spiritual meaning in pain and accept life with pain. Through prayer, one participant realized that 'one can lead a good life, despite pain'. Some of the participants equated prayer with hope. Maria surrendered herself to God, knowing with certainty that God will help her:

> 'Praying means hope...I am always hoping...you put everything in god's hands and knowing that eventually, he will listen to my prayers and knowing with certainty that I will get better.'

Carmen spends all her day in bed, feeling miserable and seems to have lost interest in everything. Prayer seems to fill an internal emotional void that nothing could replace. She desperately pleads to God to alleviate her pain:

> 'It (rosary) helps...it fills my heart (cries)...and I beg the Virgin Mary to cure me. I beg her to alleviate the pain. That is all I ask for...I don't want anything else.'

Seeking to Access Social Support Networks

Phil believes his family is everything for him. It is the thing that keeps him going: *'If I didn't have support I wouldn't be here now.'* Nonetheless, although social support was an indispensable form of coping, not all participants felt supported. For instance, when talking about his family Brian remarked: *'Sometimes they don't even let me talk about it! They just don't want to hear!'*

Futile attempts to feel understood resulted in giving up striving to maintain friendship networks. The lack of understanding created a distinction between the chronic pain sufferer and the rest of society that is oblivious to pain:

> 'People don't really worry about something unless it happens to them...so unless it happens to you...you don't really know what it feels like' (Doris)

Nonetheless, talking about pain and externalizing one's feelings was perceived as helpful.

Accessing Psychological Therapy to 'Tackle Issues'
Of the few participants who sought psychological help, those who did perceive it as 'an indispensable source of support' and a way to 'tackle issues', something they were unable to do with other health care professionals.

ACCEPTING PAIN INTO SENSE OF SELF

A possible stage in the process of coping entails acceptance. This can lead to a sense of mastery and control and to the reconstruction of a new sense of self, mostly by *adapting to a modified me*.

> 'The best approach is to make your enemy your best friend' and 'You carry pain in style. You do not struggle any more. Accepting for me means I have to carry this load and I am ok. It is not being imposed on me.' (Laura)
> 'You get used to it...you learn to live with it...imagine being born with one arm...you have to learn to do everything with the other arm...you just accept it and life goes on'. (Nick)

Acceptance is seldom a straightforward process, nor is it always the happy ending.

> 'Unfortunately, you learn to live with the pain...for me this is masochism!'(Ivan)

Acquiescing to Pain as a Stronger Force

This theme encapsulates i) retreating in one's personal world and ii) death as a possible yet unacceptable solution.

Retreating in One's Personal World
Sometimes, pain takes over, resulting in a sense of disconnectedness from the world outside, with a predominance of depressive symptoms. 'You may think I am crazy, but I'd rather have cancer!... At least I know there is an end in sight! I feel very unhappy and alone.'(Rita)

Death as a Possible Yet Unacceptable Solution
Sometimes, death is perceived as the only solution, albeit an unacceptable one. This was due to repercussions it could have on family members.

> 'Had I been separated or had I been childless, I would have contemplated an overdose...yes I would surely have committed suicide.' (Rita)

> 'It crosses my mind to grab a knife...or simply jump off the roof...I sometimes feel like taking my life'. (Doris)

Death was unacceptable also due to the perceived unacceptability of death by suicide in a Roman Catholic society:

> 'I go to the cemetery and beg and pray to them (parents) to take me with them, the pain is too much...but they won't take me. If only I could I would kill myself.'(Carmen)

THE JOURNEY TO COPING

Inter-related themes resulted in the emergence of a grounded theory model entitled *The Journey to Coping* as shown in Figure 1 below. It reflects the long process of adaptation to life with pain, revealing how potential relations of aforementioned 13 sub-themes portray a cause and effect relationship, resulting in the bridging of the final categories. Relations between categories are not necessarily sequential and predictable but irregular and fluctuating. The journey to coping is seldom smooth. Escalating pain entails repeated adaptations as individuals start experiencing new losses and decreased functioning.

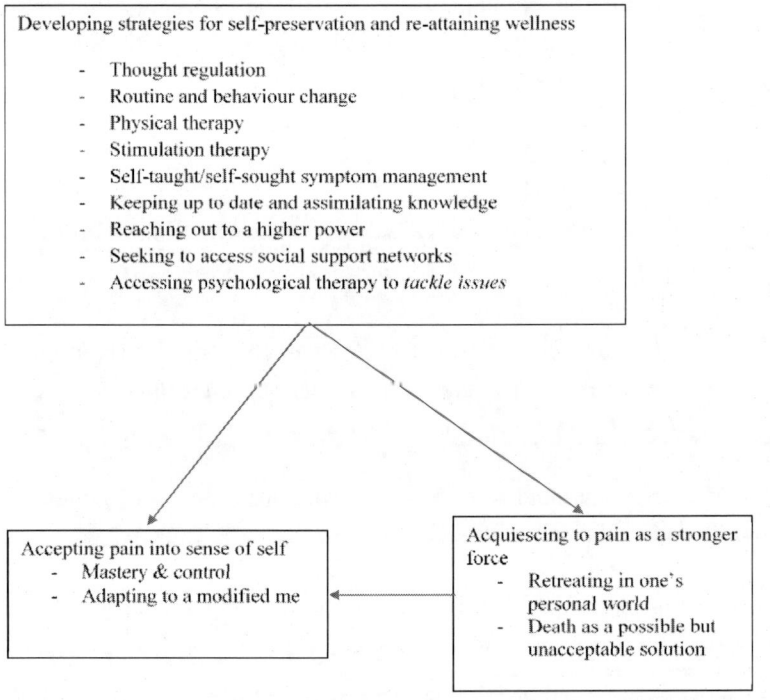

Figure 1. The Journey to Coping.

DISCUSSION

This study has shed light on specific pain coping patterns from a Maltese perspective. The emergent theory supports and extends previous literature by shedding light on the chronic pain sufferer's journey to coping with an unpleasant reality. Unlike previous research documenting high medication usage amongst chronic pain sufferers (Kerns et al. 2011), Maltese patients seem quite reluctant to rely on drug-based therapies for alleviating pain, with medicinal abuse being more pronounced amongst participants with co-morbid symptoms such as depression. Similar findings were disseminated in a study in Finland where the importance of psychiatric screening amongst chronic pain patients was highlighted (Knaster et al. 2012).

A number of techniques for self-preservation and re-attaining wellness have been identified. Findings replicate emotion and problem-focused coping strategies identified by Lazarus and Folkman (1984). While the latter included information-seeking, use of alternative therapies and behavioural interventions, the former included seeking social support, spirituality and cognitive restructuring to adapt to a newly imposed identity. Interestingly, despite some resistance to psychologically-oriented therapies, most participants were unknowingly resorting to psychological coping techniques including reframing, grounding, positivity and imagery. In accordance with previous findings, some participants seemed to have adjusted well and accepted pain, despite obvious limitations imposed (Mourão et al. 2010). Acceptance-based approaches have been linked to better functioning and decreased symptoms of anxiety and depression amongst chronic pain patients in a primary care setting in the UK (McCracken et al. 2013).

Acceptance does not mean giving up, it means letting go of the need to control pain. Ironically, letting go of the need to control pain resulted in increased mastery and control *over* pain. Within this context, control means stopping pain from interfering with one's life and letting go of unsuccessful efforts to find a cure. Participants with an internal health locus of control seemed to be coping better and displayed less anxiety than those with an external locus of control (Kupla et al. 2014). The former term reflects a personal evaluation of whether one's health is controlled by the self or external circumstances or faith (Wallston & Wallston, 1982). Participants with an external locus of control were more inclined to rely on ineffective problem-focused strategies such as bed-seeking behaviour or passivity.

Findings corroborate those identified in previous literature with Belgian chronic pain patients whereby participants who were having problems coping were finding it extremely difficult to engage in previously enjoyable activities, believing they were better off dead (Dezeutter et al. 2015). Although none had actually attempted suicide, 5 out of 21 participants reported suicidal ideation. Findings coincide with a review by Tang and Crane (2006) reporting similar statistics for the prevalence of suicidal ideation amongst chronic pain sufferers in the US. Pain intensity, helplessness, hopelessness and duration increased the risk of death by suicide. Depressive symptoms and enduring suffering render death less fearful for these patients, as exemplified in literature (Hooley et al. 2014). In line with findings of a quantitative study conducted in Canada by Wilson, Kowal, Henderson, McWilliams & Pelopuin (2013), participants with suicidal ideation were more likely to experience a sense of disconnectedness from the rest of the world. While social support was a buffer against suicide, spirituality helped foster acceptance as reported in earlier studies (Moreira-Almeida & Koenig, 2008). Nonetheless, the latter was unhelpful when it resulted in passive coping strategies and when participants resorted to higher powers to solve their problem. This can result in higher levels of psychopathology. Results from a non-linear model study reveal that the latter was higher in more frequent church attendees as opposed to individuals with moderate frequency of church attendance (O'Connell-Edwards et al. 2009). Cognitive behavior therapy (CBT) may promote active coping by modifying dysfunctional beliefs and faulty information-processing techniques, helping the individual break free from emotional helplessness and imparting an increased sense of self-efficacy to take adaptive action (Beck 1976). Self-efficacy refers to the individual's ability to perform a behavior to meet a specific positive outcome (Bandura 1977). Pain self-efficacy has been found to reduce fear-avoidance, pain-related disability and foster better pain coping (Simons & Kaczynski 2012).

Maladaptive coping skills contrast with an existential approach adopted by a few who managed to find personal meaning in pain. Man's search for meaning is a natural, healthy and motivational driving force (Frankl 1963). Individuals having the ability to connect to life values are better able to endure suffering and find a sense of purpose. Within the current context, finding meaning means finding a reason to live rather than giving in to a meaningless existence. A construction of personal meaning and purpose has been linked to a number of psychological and physical benefits including decreased pain and lower distress (Scrignaro et al. 2014).

In line with constructs from acceptance and commitment therapy (ACT), connecting with values can help overcome life challenges and fostering a meaningful life (Harris 2008). ACT promotes valued action by encouraging individuals to accept pleasant and unpleasant thoughts and sensations in a non-judgmental way, without attempting to modify them or act on them (McCracken et al. 2013). Cognitive diffusion techniques and experiential acceptance help the person develop effective coping patterns that bring them closer to their chosen values (Wilson et al. 1999).

Although the theme of *death* is not a novel construct in pain literature, what is perhaps strikingly different amongst Maltese participants was the fact that death was perceived as an unacceptable solution. Such findings reinforce the subjective and cultural perceptions of pain. Although religion seemed to be a protective factor in preventing suicide, it also seemed a major impediment to suicide. While concern regarding dishonouring family members was identified as one possible obstacle, some participants who relied on religious coping often prayed to God to take them with him. Although this theme was not always specifically stated, it was utterly implied several times. It is possible that some participants perceived suicide as sinful in the eyes of God. These fears could be particularly true in a devout nation such as Malta, where Roman Catholicism remains a trademark of Maltese culture. Apart from that, the impact death could have on one's family seemed an unforgettable sin.

Implications for Clinical Practice

Further to findings outlined above, a number of important implications have been identified. Since self-efficacy can result in increased adjustment, solution brief-focused therapy (De Shazer et al. 1986) can be one way of enhancing perceived control by facilitating meaningful life changes (Gingerich et al. 2013). Incorporating skills from SBFT can be beneficial to patients who are resorting to passive life-styles and who are struggling to make the required life changes to foster better adaptation. Individuals with an external locus of control are less inclined to adopt active coping strategies. Assessing the locus of control of potential service users may be necessary to identify the most appropriate may forward. Possibly, these individuals may benefit from more directive and prescriptive approaches to engage in the desired behaviour.

The finding that a sense of belongingness serves to outweigh feelings of perceived burdensomeness and to decrease the risk of suicide has important implications. Results put added responsibility on clinicians who have a duty to make a holistic assessment of the presenting problem, including assessing the psychological well-being of patients and a psychiatric evaluation and referring accordingly. This is particularly important since doctors are usually the first line of contact for most chronic pain patients. The assessment and treatment for depression is part of the GP training in Malta. Nonetheless, GPs may require additional training to be able to identify signs of psychological distress, particularly amongst chronic pain patients since pain is often physical in nature and the psychological aspect may be ignored by medical professionals. The possibility of additional training for doctors working in pain clinics merits consideration. Addressing the psychosocial impact of chronic pain helps ensure a holistic treatment. CBT for suicidality can help shift negative thoughts and distortions and reduce feelings of burdensomeness as identified in a qualitative study on older adults experience of pain associated with leg ulceration (Taverner et al. 2014). Incorporating constructs from dialectic behavior therapy (Linehan 1993) can foster adaptive coping and reduce self-harm in patients with suicidal ideation (Taverner et al. 2014). Since social support seems to act as a buffer to suicidality, the possibility of setting up therapist-led or self-help support groups within the local hospital merits some careful thought. Findings reinforce the need to draft a national suicide prevention strategy as identified by Xuereb (2014) in order to address existing gaps in service provision and reinforce existing ones.

Existential therapy aims to help individuals come to terms with past, present and future crisis, to widen their perspectives of the world and to foster a valuable and meaningful existence (Dryden 2007). Resolution of existential struggles is particularly beneficial in improving the overall quality of life of individuals suffering from chronic illnesses (Dezutter et al. 2015). Investigating the possibility and efficacy of incorporating existential approaches to existing pain management therapies could offer new insights to the understanding of chronic pain and coping.

The need to take into account the religious dimension in therapeutic interventions with chronic pain patients has been identified elsewhere (Rippentrop 2005). Awareness of religious coping mechanisms by health care professionals may shed light on helpful and unhelpful coping strategies and may need to be addressed in order to yield effective treatment outcomes. Health care professionals may need to liaise with religious affiliations in Malta to raise awareness of the distinct roles of each professional and to ensure a smoother referral process. Rippentrop (2005) suggests taking a religious history of clients as part of the initial assessment, with the hope of gathering important information about factors influencing prognosis for recovery. Integrating spiritual dimensions in CBT by identifying negative thoughts clients may have in relation to their situation and replacing unhealthy beliefs with more balanced and rational cognitions. Incorporating mindfulness meditation practices from a spiritual perspective may be another way of overcoming potential resistance to the uptake of psychological services. Health care professionals and chaplains who interact with individuals experiencing chronic pain may be trained to provide *autonomy support* practices to equip the sufferer with skills needed to build self-determination or the motivation to mobilize effort in order to live a more fulfilling life.

FUTURE RESEARCH

Although current findings may not necessarily be transferable to all chronic pain sufferers, they provide a research base that is sufficient enough to make a few recommendations for the holistic treatment of chronic pain. An understanding of the perspectives of health care professionals' perceptions of coping responses of chronic pain patients may provide further information and guidance regarding how to most effectively influence positive coping responses within the health care system. Since the doctor-patient interaction is an important component of pain management, clinicians' perceptions of pain and its treatment may shed some light on the delivery of existing pain services and ways of improving this. The current study was exploratory since grounded theory is a starting point for future research on pain coping. The emergent theory could be expanded upon with data from a longitudinal perspective following coping mechanisms over time. This could compare coping strategies and attitudes of participants of different ages to assist researchers to further develop emerging themes. Future research could also shed light on how pain coping may be related to key outcomes for Maltese chronic pain individuals including psychological functioning, pain-related disability and quality of life. A high sense of self-efficacy has been linked to better pain coping. Future research could seek to explore the Maltese's construction and understanding of the term and how this relates to pain coping since social, economic and cultural factors have been found to influence perceptions of self-efficacy (Burke et al. 2009).

Findings point to the need to exploit the potential of triangulation methods of data collection to capture more fully the richness and complexity of human behaviour and experience. Further theoretical sampling with individuals who are under 45 years of age may reveal differences in participants' interpretation of pain experiences, something worth investigating.

STRENGTHS AND LIMITATIONS

A number of strengths can be identified. Participants were balanced in terms of gender, making comparability experiences possible. They were all of Maltese nationality, reflecting a good picture of prevalent coping strategies amongst the Maltese population. The use of grounded theory allowed for the emergence of a new theory with an unexplored population and in-depth exploration of pain coping. A constructivist approach allows the acknowledgment of the researcher's subjectivity and meaning-making to emerge. The sample size renders generalization more possible, thereby shedding light on common coping mechanisms. Individual reality is socially constructed and a reflection of the social world which render it potentially generalisable (Willig 2001).

A number of limitations warrant acknowledgment. None of the interviewees refused to participate, possibly implying that those contacted may have had less of a supportive family environment and were therefore more willing to share their experience. Since pain duration varied, it is therefore possible that the experience of participants who had been suffering from pain for a number of years was different to those enduring a more recent onset. Some pain conditions were still undiagnosed. This uncertainty could have had a detrimental effect on pain coping strategies and distress levels. The majority of participants had a secondary level of education and were over 45 years of age, making results were more representative of this particular segment of the Maltese society. Finally, unresolved traumatic experiences endured by some participants could have influenced the pain experienced and conclusively, the coping strategies employed.

CONCLUSION

Pain coping mechanisms amongst the Maltese revolve mostly round a number of self-taught/self-sought strategies, with a seeming reluctance to rely on pharmacological treatments. Findings from this study also reveal that the journey to coping is rarely straightforward and that although some participants have adjusted well to pain, others are still struggling to accept a painful reality.

Funding

This work was partly supported by the Malta Government Scholarship Scheme.

Declaration of Conflicting Interests

The author declares no potential conflicts of interest with respect to the research, authorship, and/ or publication of this article.

References

Azzopardi Muscat, Natasha, Neville Calleja, Martin Balzan, Josie Muscat, and Catherine Calleja. "Heathcare Delivery in Malta. A Publication Outlining Trends within the Healthcare Sector." August 2018. Accessed June 25, 2019. http://www.pwc.com/en_MT/mt/publications/healthcare/assets/healthcare_delivery_august_2012.pdf.

Bandura, Albert. "Self-efficacy: toward a unifying theory of behavioral change." *Psychological Review* 84, no. 2 (1977): 191.

Beck, Aaron T. *Cognitive Therapy and the Emotional Disorders*. New York: International Universities Press, 1976.

Been, Jasper V., Jeanne P. Dieleman, Titia Katgert, Tera Boelen-van der Loo, Sylvia M. van der Pal, Monique van Dijk, Boris W. Kramer, and Peter Andriessen. "Pain coping strategies: Neonatal intensive care unit survivors in adolescence." *Early Human Development* 103 (2016): 27-32.

Birbili, Maria. "Translating from one language to another." *Social Research Update* 31, no. 1 (2000): 1-7.

Boeije, Hennie. "A purposeful approach to the constant comparative method in the analysis of qualitative interviews." *Quality and Quantity* 36, no. 4 (2002): 391-409.

Brink, Hill IL. "Validity and reliability in qualitative research." *Curationis* 16, no. 2 (1993): 35-38.

Burke, Nancy J., Joyce A. Bird, Melissa A. Clark, William Rakowski, Claudia Guerra, Judith C. Barker, and Rena J. Pasick. "Social and cultural meanings of self-efficacy." *Health Education & Behavior* 36, 5 (2009): 111S-128S.

Charmaz, Kathy. "Grounded theory: Objectivist and constructivist methods." *Handbook of Qualitative Research* 2 (2000): 509-535.

Code of Ethics of the British Psychological Society: Code of Conduct, Ethical Principles and Guidelines. (2009). Leciester: BPS.

Creswell, John W. *Qualitative Inquiry and Research Design: Choosing Among Five Traditions*. Thousand Oaks, CA: Sage Publications, 1998.

Davidhizar, R., and J. N. Giger. "A review of the literature on care of clients in pain who are culturally diverse." *International Nursing Review* 51, no. 1 (2004): 47-55.

De Shazer, Steve, Insoo Kim Berg, E. V. E. Lipchik, Elam Nunnally, Alex Molnar, Wallace Gingerich, and Michele Weiner-Davis. "Brief therapy: Focused solution development." *Family Process* 25, no. 2 (1986): 207-221.

Dey, I. *Grounding Grounded Theory: Guidelines for Qualitative Inquiry*. San Diego, CA: Academic, 1999.

Dezutter, Jessie, Koen Luyckx, and Amy Wachholtz. "Meaning in life in chronic pain patients over time: associations with pain experience and psychological well-being." *Journal of Behavioral Medicine* 38, no. 2 (2015): 384.

Dezutter, Jessie, Koen Luyckx, and Amy Wachholtz. "Meaning in life in chronic pain patients over time: associations with pain experience and psychological well-being." *Journal of Behavioral Medicine* 38, no. 2 (2015): 384-396.

Dryden, Windy, ed. *Dryden's Handbook of Individual Therapy*. SAGE, 2007.

Engel, George L. "The need for a new medical model: a challenge for biomedicine." *Science* 196, no. 4286 (1977): 129-136.

Frankl, Viktor E. "Man's Search for Meaning: An Introduction to Logotherapy." *American Journal of Orthopsychiatry* 33, no. 2 (1963): 390-390.

Gingerich, Wallace J., and Lance T. Peterson. "Effectiveness of solution-focused brief therapy: A systematic qualitative review of controlled outcome studies." *Research on Social Work Practice* 23, no. 3 (2013): 266-283.

Glaser, Barney G., Anselm L. Strauss, and Elizabeth Strutzel. "The discovery of grounded theory; strategies for qualitative research." *Nursing Research* 17, no. 4 (1968): 364.

Gouder, A. *Religious Affiliation in Malta and Gozo*. Ecclesiastical Directory Media Centre, Blata l-Bajda, Malta, 2011.

Guillemin, Marilys, and Lynn Gillam. "Ethics, reflexivity, and "ethically important moments" in research." *Qualitative Inquiry* 10, no. 2 (2004): 261-280.

Hamilton, E. S. *A grounded theory of coping among women with chronic pelvic pain* [Thesis]. California, CA, Saybrook Graduate School and Research Center (2010).

Harris, R. *The Happiness Trap: How to Stop Struggling and Start Living*. Boston: Trumpeter. 2008.

Hewstone, Miles, Antony Stephen Reid Manstead, and Wolfgang Stroebe. *The Blackwell Reader in Social Psychology*. Oxford: Blackwell, 1997.

Hiatt, John F. "Spirituality, medicine, and healing." *Southern Medical Journal* 79, no. 6 (1986): 736-743.

Hooley, Jill M., Joseph C. Franklin, and Matthew K. Nock. "Chronic pain and suicide: understanding the association." *Current Pain and Headache Reports* 18, no. 8 (2014): 435.

Kazarian, Shahe S., and David R. Evans, eds. *Handbook of Cultural Health Psychology*. New York: Oxford University Press, 2001.

Keogh, E., L. McCracken, and C. Eccleston. "Pain and gender psychosocial: Gender differences in outcome from a multidisciplinary pain management intervention." *The Journal of Pain* 5, no. 3 (2004): S99.

Kerns, Robert D., John Sellinger, and Burel R. Goodin. "Psychological treatment of chronic pain." *Annual Review of Clinical Psychology* 7 (2011): 411-434.

Knaster, Peter, Hasse Karlsson, Ann-Mari Estlander, and Eija Kalso. "Psychiatric disorders as assessed with SCID in chronic pain patients: the anxiety disorders precede the onset of pain." *General Hospital Psychiatry* 34, no. 1 (2012): 46-52.

Kulpa, Marta, Mariola Kosowicz, Beata J. Stypuła-Ciuba, and Dorota Kazalska. "Anxiety and depression, cognitive coping strategies, and health locus of control in patients with digestive system cancer." *Przeglad Gastroenterologiczny* 9, no. 6 (2014): 329.

Lam, Amy G., and Nolan WS Zane. "Ethnic differences in coping with interpersonal stressors: A test of self-construals as cultural mediators." *Journal of Cross-Cultural Psychology* 35, no. 4 (2004): 446-459.

Langdridge, Darren, and Stephanie Taylor. *Critical Readings in Social Psychology*. Milton Keynes: Open University Press, 2007.

Lazarus, Richard S., and Susan Folkman. *Stress, Appraisal, and Coping*. New York: Springer, 1984.

Linehan, Marsha. *Skills Training Manual for Treating Borderline Personality Disorder*. Vol. 29. New York: Guilford Press, 1993.

McCracken, Lance M., Ayana Sato, and Gordon J. Taylor. "A trial of a brief group-based form of acceptance and commitment therapy (ACT) for chronic pain in general practice: pilot outcome and process results." *The Journal of Pain* 14, no. 11 (2013): 1398-1406.

Meleis, Afaf Ibrahim. "Culturally competent scholarship: Substance and rigor." *Advances in Nursing Science* 19, no. 2 (1996): 1-16.

Moreira-Almeida, Alexander, and Harold G. Koenig. "Religiousness and spirituality in fibromyalgia and chronic pain patients." *Current Pain and Headache Reports* 12, no. 5 (2008): 327-332.

Mourão, Ana Filipa, Fiona M. Blyth, and Jaime C. Branco. "Generalised musculoskeletal pain syndromes." *Best Practice & Research Clinical Rheumatology* 24, no. 6 (2010): 829-840.

O'Connell-Edwards, Cara F., Christopher L. Edwards, Michele Pearce, Amy B. Wachholtz, Mary Wood, Malik Muhammad, Brittani Leach-

Beale et al. "Religious coping and pain associated with sickle cell disease: Exploration of a non-linear model." *Journal of African American Studies* 13, no. 1 (2009): 1.

Oktay, Julianne S. *Grounded Theory.* UK: Oxford University Press, 2012.

Rennie, David L., Jeffrey R. Phillips, and Georgia K. Quartaro. "Grounded Theory: A Promising Approach To Conceptualization In Psychology?." *Canadian Psychology* 29, no. 2 (1988): 139-150.

Rippentrop, A. Elizabeth. "A Review of the Role of Religion and Spirituality in Chronic Pain Populations." *Rehabilitation Psychology* 50, no. 3 (2005): 278.

Sarafino, Edward P., and Timothy W. Smith. *Health Psychology: Biopsychosocial Interactions.* USA: John Wiley & Sons, 2014.

Scrignaro, M., E. Bianchi, C. Brunelli, G. Miccinesi, C. Ripamonti, M. Magrin, and C. Borreani. "Seeking and experiencing meaning: Exploring the role of meaning in promoting mental adjustment and eudaimonic well-being in cancer patients". *Palliative and Supportive Care,* 13, no.3 (2014): 673 681.

Simons, Laura E., and Karen J. Kaczynski. "The Fear Avoidance model of chronic pain: examination for pediatric application." *The Journal of Pain* 13, no. 9 (2012): 827-835.

Strauss, Anselm, and Juliet Corbin. *Basics of Qualitative Research.* Newbury Park CA: Sage Publications, 1990.

Tang, Nicole KY, and Catherine Crane. "Suicidality in chronic pain: a review of the prevalence, risk factors and psychological links." *Psychological Medicine* 36, no. 5 (2006): 575-586.

Taverner, Tarnia, S. José Closs, and Michelle Briggs. "The journey to chronic pain: a grounded theory of older adults' experiences of pain associated with leg ulceration." *Pain Management Nursing* 15, no. 1 (2014): 186-198.

Vulliamy, Graham, Keith Lewin, and David Stephens. Doing educational research in developing countries: *Qualitative Strategies.* Routledge, 1990.

Wallston, Kenneth A., and Barbara Strudler Wallston. "Who is responsible for your health." *The Construct of Health Locus of Control in Social*

Psychology of Health and Illness. Lawrence Erlbaum Hillsdale, NJ (1982): 65-95.

Willig, Carla. *Qualitative Research in Psychology: A Practical Guide to Theory and Method.* Buckingham: Open University Press, 2001.

Wilson, K. G., S. Hayes, and K. Strosahl. *Acceptance and Commitment Therapy: An Experiential Approach to Behavior Change.* New York: Guilford Press, 1999.

Wilson, Keith G., John Kowal, Peter R. Henderson, Lachlan A. McWilliams, and Katherine Péloquin. "Chronic pain and the interpersonal theory of suicide." *Rehabilitation Psychology* 58, no. 1 (2013): 111.

Xuereb, M. (2014). *Suicide can be stopped. T.* [online] Available at: https://www.timesofmalta.com/articles/view/20140910/opinion/Suicide-can-be-stopped.535092 [Accessed 25 Jun. 2019].

In: Chronic Pain
Editor: Stefan Friedman

ISBN: 978-1-53616-296-7
© 2019 Nova Science Publishers, Inc.

Chapter 3

SELF-EMPOWERMENT, SELF-EFFICACY AND MINDFULNESS: DOES MULTIDISCIPLINARY PAIN THERAPY INHIBIT OR SUPPORT?

Michael Hartmann[*], *and Jutta Kirchner, PhD*
Pain Clinic Zurich, Zurich, Switzerland

ABSTRACT

Objectives: Today's pain management ought to be executed in a multidisciplinary and - even better - an interdisciplinary setting. Unfortunately, due to various types of discourse and different beliefs, this may lead to non-acceptance of the other party's competence and might even be judged as an offence to one's own practice.

To achieve an increase in the mutual appreciation of the somatic and the psychological perspective we address:

---

[*] Corresponding Author's E-mail: michael.hartmann@schmerz-zuerich.ch.

- the imperative need of pain-treatment for the patient who is in distress:
- the reduced interference of interventional pain management with the patient's self-empowerment compared to medical therapy with long-lasting pharmaceuticals;
- the increase of self-efficacy once the patient's "active" mode is (re-)installed; and
- methods of accepting some chronic pain using tools to remove the focus on pain from the patient's attention.

Methods: In order to also consider pain as an expression of suffering, which is an integral part of life, we have consulted philosophical sources. In order to evaluate long-term, and in particular drug therapy, pain-specific self-efficacy and mindfulness techniques, we conducted a database search (pubmed).

Results: Chronic pain and suffering have to be discussed not in a utilitarian framework but in a phenomenological context inspired by Schopenhauer, Wittgenstein, Jaspers, van Buitendijk, Scheler and Merleau-Ponty. There is an imperative need for pain-treatment for the patient who is in distress. No literature could be identified regarding whether or not interventional pain management implies reduced interference with patients' self empowerment compared to medical therapy with long-lasting pharmaceuticals. Studies on self-efficacy and those on methods of accepting some chronic pain will be discussed.

Discussion: Chronic pain, as all suffering, develops from being essential to being existential. To a certain extent, it is a contingent part of life, and it might even be meaningful. A multidisciplinary team therapy should generally be targeted at lowering the pain level to create valences for the patients, to subsequently enable them to take control again.

Keywords: interdisciplinary pain management, interventional pain management, self-empowerment, self-efficacy, mindfulness

INTRODUCTION

Today's pain management ought to be executed in a multidisciplinary and - even better - an interdisciplinary setting. Unfortunately, even in established pain clinics, therapists representing the somatic perspective and those representing the psychological perspective often live and practice in "different" worlds, due to various types of discourse, different types of education, and different beliefs. This may lead to non-acceptance of the other party's competence and might even be judged as an offence to one's own practice. We see a need for clarification and understanding in publications that highlight the synergistic effects of combining somatic and psychological therapies in pain management and thus may increase the mutual appreciation of both disciplines.

To achieve this, we address:

- the imperative need of pain-treatment for the patient who is in distress;
- the reduced interference of interventional pain management with the patient's self-empowerment compared to medical therapy with long-lasting pharmaceuticals;
- the increase of self-efficacy once the patient's "active" mode is (re-)installed; and
- methods of accepting some chronic pain using tools to remove the focus on pain from the patient's attention.

Materials and Methods: In order to also consider pain as an expression of suffering, which is an integral part of life, we have consulted philosophical sources. In order to evaluate long-term, and in particular drug therapy, pain-specific self-efficacy and mindfulness techniques, we conducted a database search (pubmed).

RESULTS

Chronic pain and suffering have to be discussed not in a utilitarian framework but in a phenomenological context inspired by Schopenhauer, Wittgenstein, Jaspers, van Buitendijk, Scheler and Merleau-Ponty. There is an imperative need for pain-treatment for the patient who is in distress. No literature could be identified on whether or not interventional pain management implies reduced interference on patients' self-empowerment compared to medical therapy with long-lasting pharmaceuticals. Studies on self-efficacy and on methods of accepting some chronic pain to a certain extent will be discussed.

DISCUSSION

Should we treat pain? Is it permissible? Should the individual do everything possible to lead a life free of pain and suffering?

As a therapist, I refer to Epicurus: "This is what it is all about: a life without pain and without fear."On the other hand, Escrivá states: "Let us bless pain. Love pain. Sanctify pain [...] – Glorify pain!"

No one can be held responsible for his/her pain; however, the attempt to take responsibility for one's pain is one of the most effective strategies in dealing with it [1].

Pain, or chronic pain, is an illness *sui generis* [2], with an unknown end and cause, which often cannot be clearly determined, and is often comprised of severe factors [3]. It is an existential threat that leaves nothing unaffected [4], resists any habituation and affirmation, narrows down time and space to endanger social relationships and communication, and will over time become normal [5; however, accepting the restructuring of the habitual body ("what I can generally do" [6]) as a new normal is rather challenging.

REACTIONS AND STRATEGIES

The experience of pain is always subjective and uncatchable [7], even though its evaluative assessment is culturally characterized [8], and communication about it is a social fact [9]. Uninvolved persons may wonder where pain goes when it appears in undulating intensity or when it is reported with a smile ("...always has a severity of 8 to 10 of 10"). May alexithymia – the inability of patients with chronic pain to express their feelings – be a reaction to their inability to share the actual pain experience with the environment without others despairing and refusing to understand or cooperate? [10] Why can everything that is important and potentially lost be the cause of pain? [11]

Other persons and therapists are hardly able to imagine the diverse dimensions that the vulnerability of the individual in pain may experience [12].

However, access to another person – and to oneself – can be found through a newly connoted shared suffering – empathy and sympathy [13]. Then, treatment of the mind and body will be targeted at supporting patients in managing their "new normal" and creating conditions in which pain can be reduced. Since chronic pain significantly inhibits the individual's motivation, self-empowerment and activity through the often-experienced despair, pain therapy should generally be targeted at lowering the pain level to create valences for the patients, to subsequently enable them to take control again via self-empowerment. This is also true when merely pain in the body – and not necessarily suffering in the perceiving body –, can be treated [14].

For this, the entire arsenal that is available to us today must be offered and used – regardless of specialist discipline.

RISK OF UNDERMINING PATIENTS' AUTONOMY

Medical interventions, i.e., therapies, that address identified somatic causes and neurophysiological/neuropathological targets, generally run the risk of undermining patients' autonomy and their participation in the process. This is all the more sustained the longer such therapies last. Interventional, minimally-invasive, and invasive therapies are, due to the limited area of their application, less intrusive than, for example, long-term medication, which also often comes with prolonged adverse effects that limit quality of life. We hypothesize that minimally-invasive pain-treatment procedures, by interfering for a shorter period of time, have less impact on patients' self-empowerment.

Cognitive and physical impairment after application of minimally-invasive pain-treatments, like infiltrations and neuroablative procedures, are rare. In contrast, oral and transdermal opioid treatment for non-malignant pain must be questioned due to the consecutive danger of falling and potentially lethal risks, such as sleep apnoea and the risk of abuse [15-17; however, many prescribing physicians and key opinion leaders consider this therapy adequate. Guidelines, for example, do not generally exclude opioid prescription in excess of six months for non-malignant pain [18].

Interventional pain-therapy procedures have a bad reputation, for example, in the German-speaking literature, and are thought to cause potentially chronic states compared with medication [19;however, the exclusively temporary influence on the patient that is inherent in many diagnostic and therapeutic interventions is not sufficiently considered in addition to these shortcomings.

FOLLOWING THERAPY: SELF-EFFICACY AND MINDFULNESS

There is no doubt that the reduction of pain is ethically justified. In the best case of partial pain reduction, treatment of the mind and body can support patients in recognizing and accepting pain as such and the resulting suffering to a certain extent – as an expression of their being alive, enabling them to push pain from the focus of their attention. Methods that support the conviction of perceived self-efficacy are important aids in this process.

Perceived self-efficacy is trust in being able to master difficult situations with your own ability [20]. Meta analyses have shown that an increase of this trust can reduce pain, for example, in arthritis, and can reduce the fear caused by tumour pain [21]. Coping strategies and physical activity can also be improved [22].

However, weak confidence in self-efficacy, as well as low social support, may lead to depression [23] – and thus, similar to increased fear avoidance – increased invalidity [24].

An active attempt can now be made to push the remaining pain, which should likely be accepted as "being part of oneself," from the focus of attention. This can be done with techniques aligned with mindfulness.

Mindfulness-based techniques that are relevant in pain medicine are derived from meditative approaches, such as MBSR (Mindfulness-Based Stress Reduction), MBCT (Mindfulness- Based Cognitive Therapy) and Zen meditation.

The first study on the secular, non-esoteric mindfulness technique MBSR for chronic pain was published by Kabat-Zinn in 1982 [25]. Its efficacy in treating chronic pelvic pain [26], the adverse effects of HIV therapy [27], fibromyalgia [28], and anxiety [29] have since been proven.

Mindfulness-based techniques can reduce pain [30] and can be effective against depression [31]. Empathy-relevant areas in the brain show increased activity both for experienced pain and when perceiving the pain of others in functional imaging in persons experienced in meditation [32, 33]. Pain is perceived as less unpleasant as a consequence [34] and resources can be activated more successfully.

Meta-analyses show "limited evidence" for their effect on acceptance, "inconclusive evidence" for their pain-reducing effect [35], and "moderate evidence" for their efficacy in treating anxiety, depression, and pain [36]. The treatment effect can be increased by (self-) hypnosis [37].

Meditation and self-hypnosis can be considered non-invasive neuromodulation methods [38].

Mindfulness-based methods are intended to support meeting pain with understanding [39], rather than avoiding or rejecting it. Such access may also increase psychological flexibility [40], as analyses of pain-diary entries suggest [41].

Mindfulness-based techniques lead to better results in groups than in individual therapy [42]. It must be noted that, to date, studies on mindfulness-based techniques have rarely been performed with an active control group [43].

PERSPECTIVE

Treatment expectations and hope for healing are important mechanisms in pain treatment.

After treatment by an empathetic therapeutic team has achieved some initial success, the further process relies on an active patient. A change of perspective may support patients in recovering their active role. In such a context, pain is not only an expression and cause of suffering, but usually also a problem for the sufferer. While managing suffering is targeted at mitigation, addressing problems requires a solution. Such a change of perspective challenges the entire emotional and intellectual creativity of the suffering person – not only for "better handling of pain" or "good pain management," but also for a conscious life design that allots pain the space in life that it is due.

REFERENCES

[1] Grüny, C. *Zerstörte Erfahrung* [*Destroyed Perception*]. Würzburg: Königshausen und Neumann, 2004.

[2] Tanner, J. Zur "Kulturgeschichte des Schmerzes." [On the Cultural History of Pain]. In: Schönbächler, G, ed. *Schmerz. Perspektiven auf eine menschliche Grunderfahrung.* Zurich: Chronos, 2007.

[3] L'evinas, E. "Das sinnlose Leiden" [Futile Suffering]. In: *Zwischen uns. Versuche über das Denken an den*. Munich, Vienna: Hanser, 1995.

[4] Garro, L.C. "Chronic Illness and the Construction of Narratives." In: Del Veccio Good MJ, ed. *Pain as a Human Experience*. Berkeley: University of California Press, 1994.

[5] Wendell S. *The Rejected Body*. New York: Routledge, 1996.

[6] Merleau-Ponty, M. *Phänomenologie der Wahrnehmung* [*Phenomenology of Perception*]. Berlin: De Gruyter, 1966.

[7] Good, B.J. "A Body in Pain – the Making of a World of Chronic Pain. In: Del Veccio and M.J. Good, eds. *Pain as Human Experience.* Berkeley:: University of California Press, 1994.

[8] Schönbächler, G. "Schmerzperspektiven" ["Perspectives of Pain"]. In: Schönbächler, G., ed. *Schmerz. Perspektiven auf eine menschliche Grunderfahrung.* Zurich: Chronos, 2007.

[9] Wittgenstein L. *Philosophische Untersuchungen* [*Philosophical Investigations*]. Oxford: Blackwell, 1958.

[10] Müller-Busch, H.C. "Soziokulturelle Aspekte des Schmerzes" ["The Socio-cultural Aspects of pPin"]. In: Bach, M., M. Aigner, and B.Bankier, eds. *Schmerzen ohne Ursache – Schmerzen ohne Ende.* Vienna: Facultas, 2001.

[11] Grüny, C. *Zerstörte Erfahrung* [*Destroyed Perception*]. Würzburg: Königshausen und Neumann, 2004.

[12] Scheler, M. *Der Formalismus in der Ethik und die Materielle Wertethik* [*Formalism in Ethics and the Material Ethics of Values*]. Bern: Francke, 1966.

[13] Grüny, C. *Zerstörte Erfahrung* [*Destroyed Perception*]. Würzburg: Königshausen und Neumann, 2004.

[14] Hell, D. "Schmerz und Leiden – Körper und Seele" ["Pain and Suffering –Body and Soul"]. In: Schönbächler, G, ed. *Schmerz. Perspektiven auf eine Menschliche Grunderfahrung.* Zurich: Chronos, 2007.

[15] Ping, F., Y.Wand, J.Wang, et al. "Opioids Increase Hip Fracture Risk: a Meta-analysis. *J. Bone Miner. Metab.* 2016 Mar. 29.

[16] Ray, W.A., C.P.Chung, K.T. Murray, K. Hall, and C.M.Stein. "Prescription of Long-acting Opiods and Mortality in Patients with Chronic Non-cancer Pain." *JAMA* 14 Jun. 2016: (22) 315;(22)415-23.

[17] Hartrick, C.T. "Editorial Note: The Opioid Epidemic: Root Cause Analysis." *Pain Pract.* 2016:(16) 787.

[18] Häuser, W., F. Bock, P. Engeser, et al. „ Recommendations of the Updated LONTS Guidelines: Long-term Opioid Therapy for Chronic Noncancer Pain." *Schmerz* [*Pain*] 2015 Feb.: 29(1):109-30.

[19] "*Kerncurriculum Schmerztherapie für die Lehre für ein Querschnittsfach Schmerztherapie nach der neuen AO*" ["*Pain therapy Core Curriculum for Teaching a Cross-sectional Subject Pain Therapy According to the New AO*"]. DGSS. Available at: http://www.dgss.org. Accessed 10 May 2016.

[20] Bandura, A. *Self-efficacy. The Exercise of Control.* New York: Freeman: 1997.

[21] Mystakidou, K., E. Tsilika, E. Parpa, I. Panagiotou A. Galanos, and A. Gouliamos. "Caregivers' Anxiety and Self-Efficacy in Palliative Care. *Eur. J. Cancer Care* (Engl). Mar. 2013: 22(2): 188-95.

[22] Sperber, N., K.S.Hall,, K. Allen, B.M. DeVellis, M.Lewis, and L.F. Callahan. "The Role of Symptoms and Self-efficacy in Predicting Physical Activity Change among Older Adults with Arthritis." *J. Phys. Act. Health* Mar. 2014: 11(3); 528-35.

[23] Pjanic, I., N. Messerli-Bürgy, M.S. Bachmann, F. Siegenthaler, U. Hoffmann-Richter, and H. Znoi H. "Predictors of Depressed Mood 12 Months after Injury: Contribution of Self efficacy and Social Support." *Disabil. Rehabil.* 2014(365): 1258-63.

[24] de Moraes Vieira, E.B., M. de Góes Salvetti,L.P. Damiani, and C.A. de Mattos Pimenta. "Self-efficacy and Fear Avoidance Beliefs in Chronic Low Back Pain Patients: Coexistence and Associated Factors." *Pain Manag. Nurs. Sept.* 2014 (15.3): 593-602.

[25] Kabat-Zinn, J. "An Outpatient Program in Behavioral Medicine for Chronic Pain Patients Based on the Practice of Mindfulness Meditation: Theoretical Considerations and Preliminary Results." *Gen. Hosp. Psychiatry* Apr. 1982 (4.1):33-47.

[26] Fox, S.D., E. Flynn, and R.H. Allen. "Mindfulness Meditation for Women with Chronic Pelvic Pain: a Pilot Study." *J. Reprod. Med.* Mar-Apr. 2011 (56.3-4): 158-162.

[27] Duncan, L.G., J.T. Moskowitz, T.B. Neilands, S.E. Dilworth, F.M. Hecht, and M. O. Johnson. "Mindfulness-based Stress Reduction for HIV Treatment Side Effects: a Randomized, Wait-list Controlled Trial." *J. Pain Symptom Manage*. Feb. 2012 (43.2): 161-71.

[28] Kozasa, E.H., L.H. Tanaka, C. Monson, C, S. Little, F.C. Leao, and M.P.Peres. "The Effects of Meditation-based Interventions on the Treatment of Fibromyalgia." *Curr. Pain Headache Rep.* Oct. 2012 (16.5): 383-7.

[29] Marchand, W.R. "Mindfulness-based Stress Reduction, Mindfulness-based Cognitive Therapy, and Zen Meditation for Depression, Anxiety, Pain, and Psychological Distress." *J. Psychiatr. Pract.* Jul. 2012 (18.4): 233-52.

[30] Reiner, K., L. Tibi, and J.D. Lipsitz. "Do Mindfulness-based Interventions Reduce Pain Intensity? A Critical Review of the Literature." *Pain Med.* Feb. 2013 (14.2): 230-42.

[31] Marchand, W.R. "Mindfulness-based Stress Reduction, Mindfulness-based Cognitive Therapy, and Zen Meditation for Depression, Anxiety, Pain, and Psychological Distress. *J. Psychiatr. Pract.* Jul. 2012 (18.4): 233-52.

[32] Mascaro, J.S., J.K.Rilling, L.T. Negi, and C.L. Raison "Pre-existing Brain Function Predicts Subsequent Practice of Mindfulness and Compassion Meditation." *Neuroimage.* 1 Apr. 2013(69): 35-42.

[33] Lutz, A., D.R. McFarlin, D.M. Perlman, T.V. Salomons, and R. J. Davidson. "Altered Anterior Insula Activation during Anticipation and Experience of Painful Stimuli in Expert Meditators." *Neuroimage.* 1 Jan. 3013 (64): 538-46.

[34] Wiedemann, J., T. Gard, B.K. Hölzel, et. al., Pain Attenuation through Mindfulness Is Associated with Decreased Cognitive Control and Increased Sensory Processing in the Brain." *Deutsche Zeitschrift für Akupunktur [German Journal for Acupuncture].* 2012 (55.2): 25-6.

[35] Cramer, H., H. Haller, R. Lauche, and G. Dobos "Mindfulness-based Stress Reduction for Low Back Pain: A Systematic Review." *BMC Complement Altern Med.* 25 Sep. 2012(12): 162.

[36] Goyal, M., S. Singh, E.M. Sibinga, et al. "Meditation Programs for Psychological Stress and Well-being: a Systematic Review and Meta-analysis." *JAMA Intern. Med.* Mar, 2014 (174.3): 357-68.

[37] Donatone, B. "Focused Suggestion with Somatic Anchoring Technique: Rapid Self-hypnosis for Pain Management." *Am. J. Clin. Hypn.* Apr. 2013 (55.4): 325-42.
[38] Jensen, M.P., M.A. Day and J. Miró. "Neuromodulatory Treatments for Chronic Pain: Efficacy and Mechanisms." *Nat. Rev. Neurol.* Mar. 2014 (10.3): 167-78.
[39] Fabbro, F. and C. Crescentini. "Facing the Experience of Pain: a Neuropsychological Perspective." *Phys. Life Rev*. Sep. 2014(11.3): 540-52.
[40] McCracken, L.M. and S.C. Velleman. "Psychological Flexibility in Adults with Chronic Pain: a Study of Acceptance, Mindfulness, and Values-based Action in Primary Care." *Pain* Jan. 2019(148.1): 141-7.
[41] Morone, N.E., C.S. Lynch, C.M. Greco, H.A. Tindle, and D.K. Weiner. "'I Felt Like a New Person': The Effects of Mindfulness Meditation on Older Adults with Chronic Pain: Qualitative Marrative Analysis of Diary Entries." *J. Pain* Sept. 2008 (9.9): 841-8.
[42] Hassed, C. "Mind body Therapies Use in Chronic Pain Management." *Aust. Fam. Physician* Mar. 2013 (42.3): 112-17.
[43] McCoon, D.G., Z.E. Imel, M.A. Rosenkranz, et al. „The Validation of an Active Control Intervention for Mindfulness Based Stress Reduction (MBSR)." *Behav. Res. Ther. Jan.* 2012 (50.1): 3-12.

BIOGRAPHICAL SKETCH

Michael Hartmann

Affiliation: Pain Clinic Zurich. Founder

Education:
Anesthesiology
Delegated Psychology
Intensive Care Medicine

Business Address: Wallisellenstrasse 301a, 8050 Zurich, Switzerland

Research and Professional Experience:
Multidisciplinary Pain Management
Interventional Pain Medicine
Ventilator-associated Pneumonia
Alpha-2-Agonists

Professional Appointments:
WIP examiner
Board Member: Swiss Society for Interventional Pain Medicine
Councillor: Swiss Society for the Study of Pain

Publications from the Last 3 Years:
Hartmann M and Baetscher A. "Analgosedation for Interventional Procedures in Patients with Acute and Chronic Pain." *Pain Pract*. Apr. 2017 (17.4):566-567. doi: 10.1111/papr.12553. Epub 3 Mar.2017.

In: Chronic Pain
Editor: Stefan Friedman

ISBN: 978-1-53616-296-7
© 2019 Nova Science Publishers, Inc.

Chapter 4

INSURERS SAVE WHILE PATIENTS PAY: THE REDISTRIBUTION OF MEDICATION COSTS FOLLOWING ENROLLMENT IN A STATE-LEGAL MEDICAL CANNABIS PROGRAM

Sarah S. Stith[1],*, PhD, Jacob M. Vigil[2], PhD, Ian Adams[3] and Anthony P. Reeve[3]

[1]Department of Economics, University of New Mexico,
Albuquerque, NM, US
[2]Department of Psychology, University of New Mexico,
Albuquerque, NM, US
[3]Industrial Rehabilitation Clinics, Albuquerque, NM, US

---

* Corresponding Author's E-mail: ssstith@unm.edu.

Abstract

State-level analyses have found prescription cost savings associated with the legalization of medical cannabis, yet little is known about how patient-level shifts in conventional medication use lead to aggregate cost savings and how they compare to medical cannabis costs. We analyze 3,434 scheduled prescription drug records for 94 chronic back pain patients from a single clinic, comparing 52 patients enrolled in the New Mexico Medical Cannabis Program (MCP) with 42 non-enrolled patients over a 24-month period. We calculate adjusted costs to insurers and patients based on average wholesale prices, dispensing fees, and patient copays and use a difference-in-differences fixed effects panel regression approach to study the association between MCP enrollment and conventional prescription drug costs. Cannabis costs are based on patient survey responses. Relative to pre-enrollment or our comparison group, MCP-enrolled patients' conventional prescriptions cost almost $200 less to insurers per month and $30 less out-of-pocket to patients at 18 months post-enrollment. With monthly medical cannabis costs of $141 (SD=$91), patients faced higher out-of-pocket costs than they did prior to enrollment in the MCP, suggesting a strong preference for cannabis. From a total cost perspective, combined insurer and patient cost savings on conventional prescriptions outweigh the costs of medical cannabis after 11 months post-enrollment in the MCP.

Keywords: pain, health insurance, pharmacoeconomic, cannabis, marijuana, opioid

1. Introduction

Healthcare costs and productivity losses associated with chronic pain conditions in the U.S. exceed those of all other major diagnoses, including cardiovascular disease, neoplasms, injury and poisoning, and endocrine, nutritional, metabolic and digestive diseases [1]. This burden is compounded by the use of, in particular, opioid medications, due to the prevalence and severity of their adverse side effects [2], rates of misuse [3, 4], risk of overdose [5, 6] and interactions with other medications [7]. Despite these costs, we know little about the costs of chronic pain treatments other than opioids and how patients choose among different therapies, including medical cannabis.

The state-level legalization of cannabis for treatment of chronic pain throughout the U.S. underscores the need for understanding how cannabis treatment affects the cost of treating chronic pain for both insurers and patients. With the exception of a few litigated workers compensation claims, no insurer covers medical cannabis meaning that the costs of medical cannabis fall entirely on patients unlike the costs of conventional prescription medications. In other words, insurers may benefit if patients switch from prescription medications to medical cannabis, while patients are likely to switch to medical cannabis only if the relative benefits outweigh the costs of obtaining medical cannabis and any negative side effects associated with its use relative to those associated with prescription medications. Aggregate state-level analyses have shown reductions in Medicare and Medicaid costs [8, 9] and opioid-related deaths in association with medical marijuana legalization [10-12] suggesting that some people, who would otherwise be using opioids (either legally or illegally), are now using medical cannabis. Our own prior research shows that enrollment in a medical marijuana program is associated with a reduction in the daily dose of opioids consumed [13] and the number of Schedule II-IV prescriptions overall [14], similar to a prospective open-label cohort study conducted in Israel [15] and larger sample survey-based studies [16].

The current investigation is the first patient-level analysis in the literature to measure changes in costs faced by providers and patients associated with legal concurrent access to medical cannabis and conventional pharmaceutical medications. Based on previous research suggesting that patients substitute medical cannabis for prescription opioids, we hypothesized that when compared to non-cannabis-using patients, enrollees in a state-authorized Medical Cannabis Program (MCP) will cost less to insurers, but that for patients, the out-of-pocket costs of medical cannabis will outweigh the cost savings associated with reduced use of conventional prescription medications. Although a shift towards patients paying for their own treatment saves insurers money, from a societal or total cost perspective, it is unclear a priori whether treating chronic pain with opioids will result in higher costs to healthcare payers than would treating chronic pain with cannabis.

2. METHODS

We conducted a retrospective, observational cohort study, approved by the Institutional Review Board at the University of New Mexico, and used a difference-in-differences fixed effects panel regression framework to evaluate the association between enrollment in the New Mexico MCP and medication costs faced by patients and insurers. The study took place at a single-physician rehabilitation clinic that provides all eligible patients the opportunity to enroll in the MCP in line with its mission of treating palliative conditions through patient education and self-management of available treatment options. While enrolled in the MCP, patients were not provided any direct medical supervision over their cannabis use nor explicitly instructed to adjust their prescription medication usage.

A convenience sample of patients, who enrolled in the MCP between 2010 and 2015, completed an informal survey one year following enrollment regarding their experiences with the MCP. In order to focus our analysis on the cost savings associated with a specific diagnosis and to facilitate selection of a comparison group, we included only surveyed MCP patients with the most commonly diagnosed condition in our sample, chronic back pain, and who filled at least one scheduled prescription in New Mexico during the first six months of our two-year sample period. The comparison group was selected from patients meeting these criteria, who visited the same clinic during the period in which the lead physician offered all his chronic back pain patients the opportunity to enroll in the MCP. To be included in the comparison group, patients must have verbally rejected of an offer of referral to the MCP and have shown no evidence of cannabis use during the period of observation as measured by biannual random urine analyses. Our study sample included 52 MCP patients (1,864 prescriptions) and 42 comparison group patients (1,370 prescriptions), which we collapsed into patient-month level counts of 1,220 and 1,008 for the MCP and comparison groups, respectively. Due to more recent MCP enrollment dates, 20 MCP patients did not have a full 18 months post-enrollment. (One patient had 12 months, one 13, one 15, two 16, and 15 were observed for 17 months.) Prescription dates for our sample range from 4/1/2010 through 12/21/2016. The first dispensary in New Mexico opened in 2009 in Albuquerque, New Mexico, the same city in which the clinic is located, meaning all MCP enrollees had access to the wide range of cannabis products allowed under New Mexico law.

In order to calculate costs to insurers, we retrieved the per-pill Average Wholesale Price (AWP) as reported by [17] for each prescription. Because the AWP is not typically the actual price paid by insurers [18,19], we adjust the AWP-based prescription cost to the negotiated price paid by New Mexico's Medicaid Program in 2017, or 86% of the AWP plus a $3.65 per prescription dispensing fee, which falls within the estimates for a range of types of insurers [19, 20]. Commercial insurers covered 48% of the prescriptions in our sample, while the rest of the prescriptions were paid for with cash (9%), Medicaid (5%), Medicare (10%), or Workers Compensation (12%). Sixty-five percent of our sample used more than one payment source during the sample period.

For costs to patients, we used the unadjusted AWP for any out-of-pocket payments because patients are generally not able to negotiate prices. We also used insurer type-specific per prescription copayment of $5 for Medicaid, $40 for Medicare and Commercial insurers, and $0 for Workers Compensation. New Mexico Medicaid recipients typically pay $5, while $40 falls in the mid-range for copayments charged by commercial insurers [21] and Medicare [22]. Workers compensation insurance in New Mexico does not charge recipients copayments. In order to estimate the cost of cannabis, we used monthly costs from survey respondents. This variable was only included in later versions of the survey leaving us with responses from only 26 of the 52 MCP patients included in this study. Therefore, we do not include cannabis costs in our outcome variables, choosing instead to focus on the more accurately measured prescription costs and then comparing these estimated outcomes to the estimated costs of cannabis. We also provide summary information on cannabis costs reported by the New Mexico Department of Health, which averaged $11.17 per gram between 07/2014 (the first period price information was available) and 12/2016. (See Supplemental Appendix Figure SA1.) After calculating the prescription-level costs, we aggregated the total prescription costs by month for each patient, summing over prescriptions filled in that month, taking into account both per pill (AWP-based) and per prescription costs (dispensing fees and copayments).

Table 1. Descriptive Statistics for Calculated Costs to Insurers and Patients

Variable	Obs	Mean	Std. Dev.	Min	Max
Monthly Costs to Insurers	2228	$ 230.00	$ 395.23	$ -	$ 4,111.03
Medicaid	2228	$ 20.02	$ 110.91	$ -	$ 1,530.53
Medicare	2228	$ 20.59	$ 132.42	$ -	$ 2,490.96
Commercial	2228	$ 138.10	$ 333.88	$ -	$ 4,111.03
Workers Compensation	2228	$ 23.91	$ 117.97	$ -	$ 2,085.60
Monthly Opioid Costs to Insurers	2228	$ 152.92	$ 321.47	$ -	$ 4,107.03
Monthly Costs to Patients	2228	$ 52.68	$ 139.42	$ -	$ 2,361.60
Out-of-pocket	2228	$ 23.80	$ 133.38	$ -	$ 2,361.60
Medicaid	2228	$ 0.32	$ 1.55	$ -	$ 20.00
Medicare	2228	$ 4.76	$ 20.86	$ -	$ 240.00
Commercial	2228	$ 23.81	$ 38.87	$ -	$ 280.00
Monthly Opioid Costs to Patients	2228	$ 29.79	$ 108.11	$ -	$ 2,361.60
Cannabis Costs - Mean	602	$ 141.17	$ 91.22	$ 10.00	$ 350.00
Cannabis Costs - 25th Percentile		$ 80.00			
Cannabis Costs - 75th Percentile		$ 240.00			
Maximum Cannabis Costs under NM law		$ 844.45			

Abbreviations: New Mexico (NM)
Notes: Data are patient-month level.

Table 1 shows descriptive statistics for our calculated outcome variables. (Descriptive Statistics for the unadjusted prescription costs priced at the AWP and the number of prescriptions are available in Supplemental Appendix Table SA1.) On average, insurers paid $230 (0.86*AWP+$3.65*number of prescriptions) per month on patients in the sample, with the commercial payers paying the largest portion. Opioid costs accounted for more than half the monthly cost at $153. Patients paid $52.68 in combined out-of-pocket and copayment costs (out-of-pocket prescription purchases+$5*number of Medicaid prescriptions+$40*number of Medicare and Commercial insurance-covered prescriptions), with the majority of the cost again accounted for by opioid medications. Average cannabis costs per month among the surveyed patients were $141, although New Mexico allows for purchases of cannabis valued at $844 per month (8 ounces over three months at $11.17 per gram).

We first compare conventional prescription costs between MCP and non-enrolled patients during the first six months and during the last six months and between the first and last six months for each group of patients separately using t-tests. We then use a difference-in-differences fixed effects panel regression approach to model the relationship between conventional prescription costs to insurers and patients using the following regression model:

$$Costs_{it} = \alpha + \beta_1 MCP_i + \beta_2 Trend1_t + \beta_3 Trend2_t + \beta_3 MCP_{it} * Trend1_t + \beta_4 MCP_{it} * Trend2_t + \gamma_i + \varepsilon_{it}$$

where costs are measured for patient i in month t, *MCP* donates enrollment status for patient i in month t, *Trend1* is a linear trend during the first six months and zero otherwise, and *Trend2* is a linear trend during the latter 18 months (post-enrollment for the MCP patients). We also include patient fixed effects to control for time-invariant patient characteristics. (Including the patient-level fixed effects washes out the main effect of MCP group designation, leaving only the interaction of MCP and the two linear trends.) Standard errors are clustered at the patient level to control for arbitrary correlation and heteroskedasticity.

In addition to the costs to insurers overall, we conduct our analyses for each insurer type (Medicaid, Medicare, Commercial, and Workers Compensation) and for opioid prescriptions only. We also conduct robustness checks for our insurer and patient cost results using random effects models and omitting MCP patients with censored observation periods (fewer than 18 months of post-MCP enrollment data).

3. RESULTS

Table 2 compares the conventional prescription costs between the first and last six months for the MCP group and between the MCP (Panel A) and comparison group during the last six months (Panel B). The simple t-test results in Panel A show that MCP patients are less costly to insurers during the last six months than they were in the first six, both overall and for opioid medications only. Patient costs for conventional prescriptions are not statistically significantly lower in the last six months of observation than they were in the first. Comparing across groups during the last six months in Panel B indicates that MCP patients had lower costs to insurers and patients than the comparison group, both overall and for opioid medications. (As shown in Supplemental Table SA2 and supporting the validity of our comparison group, no statistically significant differences exist between the comparison and MCP groups during the first six months in terms of insurer and patient costs overall or for opioids specifically (Panel A), and costs to insurers and patients are not statistically significantly different between first and last six months in the comparison group (Panel B)).

Our regression results are presented in Table 3 show that overall trends in costs to insurers and patients are statistically insignificant throughout the observation period. The interaction between (future) MCP enrollment and the trend in period 1 (months 1 to 6) is statistically insignificant, supporting our common trends assumption. The association between MCP enrollment and costs is clear for insurers in the second period; among the MCP group of patients monthly insurer costs trend downward with a coefficient of -

$11.08 (p<0.001) in the second period (months 7 to 24). In other words, patients cost $110.80 less in the tenth month post-enrollment than they did at the time of enrollment. Opioid costs account for much of the difference and are $73.22 less in the tenth month than they were at the time of enrollment. Monthly costs to patients trend downward with a coefficient of -$1.67 (p<0.10), but the decrease is statistically insignificant for opioid prescriptions alone. (Results from random effects regressions are essentially identical as shown in Supplemental Appendix SA3-5).

Table 2. Comparing MCP Costs during the 1st and Last Six Months and across Patient Groups in the Last Six Months

Panel A: MCP Only - First v. Last Six Months			
	1st Six Months	Last Six Months	P Value
Monthly Costs to Insurers	250.53	163.27	<0.001
Monthly Opioid Costs to Insurers	186.54	102.94	<0.001
Monthly Costs to Patients	43.28	44.45	0.876
Monthly Opioid Costs to Patients	17.50	15.50	0.384
Panel B: Group Contrast - Last Six Months			
	Comparison	MCP	P Value
Monthly Costs to Insurers	282.23	163.27	<0.001
Monthly Opioid Costs to Insurers	184.09	102.94	<0.001
Monthly Costs to Patients	65.90	44.45	0.002
Monthly Opioid Costs to Patients	49.54	15.50	<0.001

Abbreviations: New Mexico Medical Cannabis Program (MCP)
Notes: P-values correspond to two-sided t-tests for continuous variables and chi-squared tests for dichotomous variables.

Figure 1 depicts the results for insurers graphically and includes the costs of cannabis. Predicted monthly costs to insurers for the comparison and the MCP group are overlaid on scatter plots of the monthly mean prescription cost in the raw data. The comparison group appears to follow a trend with essentially a zero slope, while the MCP group shows a clear downward trend in the second period with the linear trend well-fitted to the underlying data. The only potential outlier is Month 19, the month just following annual MCP license renewal, suggesting patients may be using the referral visit as an opportunity to renew conventional prescription medications as well.

Table 3. Regressions of Monthly Costs to Insurers and Patients on MCP Enrollment

Outcome ($)	(1) Costs to Insurers	(2) Costs to Patients	(3) Opioid Costs to Insurers	(4) Opioid Costs to Patients
Trend 1	-6.987	-0.445	-5.031	0.699
	(7.673)	(2.027)	(5.738)	(1.653)
MCP * Trend 1	11.36	2.269	2.299	-0.473
	(11.27)	(2.397)	(9.199)	(1.749)
Trend 2	0.718	1.065	0.309	0.665
	(2.140)	(0.739)	(1.342)	(0.618)
MCP * Trend 2	-11.08***	-1.661*	-7.322***	-0.836
	(3.539)	(0.942)	(2.345)	(0.672)
Patient-Month Observations	2,228	2,228	2,228	2,228
R-squared	0.022	0.002	0.017	0.001
Number of Patients	94	94	94	94

Abbreviations: New Mexico Medical Cannabis Program (MCP).

Notes: Each column represents a separate regression. The regressions in Columns (3) and (4) replicate the regressions in Columns (1) and (2) including only opioid prescription-related costs in the outcome variables. Individual patient fixed effects are included with standard errors are clustered at the patient level and reported in parentheses. * p<0.01, **p<0.05, *** p<0.01.

Table 4 splits out the costs by payer. Note that patients often use more than one payer, so these are not separate samples of patients, i.e., the insurer designation is based on who paid for the prescription. Overall period-level trends and the differential MCP trend in the first period are statistically insignificant. In the second period, MCP participation is associated with decreasing costs to Medicaid of -$2.05 (p<0.05) each month post-enrollment and to commercial insurers of -$5.06 (p<0.1) each month. For patients the differences are also driven by Medicaid and commercially covered prescriptions with patients' payments trending down -$0.02 each month (p<0.10) for Medicaid-covered prescriptions and -$0.89 (p<0.05) for commercially covered prescriptions during the months post-enrollment.

Table 4. Monthly Costs to Individual Insurers

Panel A: Costs to Individual Insurer Types				
Insurance Type:	Medicaid	Medicare	Commercial	Workers Compensation
Trend 1	1.622	0.681	-6.999	0.0159
	(1.856)	(0.513)	(7.083)	(1.939)
MCP*Trend 1	-3.949	0.840	10.740	0.168
	(2.524)	(3.700)	(10.35)	(2.104)
Trend 2	-0.000	-0.177	1.001	0.428
	(0.226)	(0.155)	(1.656)	(1.075)
MCP*Trend 2	-2.05**	0.203	-5.056*	-0.959
	(0.920)	(1.200)	(2.728)	(1.124)
R-squared - Within	0.019	0.001	0.005	0.001
Panel B: Costs to Patients by Insurer Type				
Insurance Type:	Patient Out-of-Pocket	Medicaid	Medicare	Commercial
Trend 1	0.08	-0.009	0.207	-0.723
	(2.014)	-0.057	(0.148)	(0.777)
MCP*Trend 1	0.583	-0.067	0.722	1.256
	(2.222)	-0.068	(0.468)	(1.158)
Trend 2	0.756	0.000	-0.018	0.327
	(0.701)	-0.007	(0.0361)	(0.284)
MCP*Trend 2	-0.956	-0.023*	-0.023	-0.891**
	(0.811)	-0.013	(0.170)	(0.426)
R-squared - Within	0.001	0.022	0.008	0.007
Observations	2,228	2,228	2,228	2,228
Number of Patients	94	94	94	94

Abbreviations: New Mexico Medical Cannabis Program (MCP).

Notes: Each column represents a separate regression for prescription costs associated with each payer type. Individual patient fixed effects are included with standard errors clustered at the patient level and reported in parentheses. * $p<0.01$, ** $p<0.05$, *** $p<0.01$.

As a sensitivity check, we also ran our regressions including only MCP patients without censored observations and finding even stronger results as show in Supplemental Appendix Table SA6.

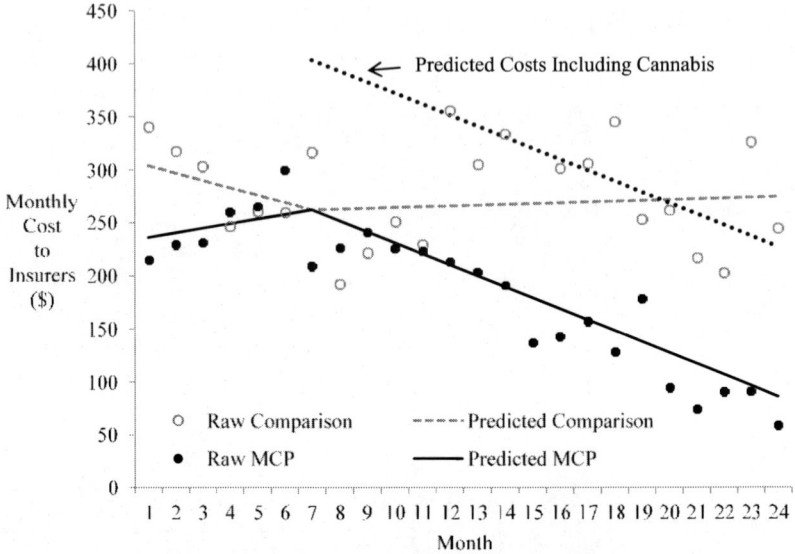

Abbreviations: New Mexico Medical Cannabis Program (MCP)
Notes: Predicted values are based on the regressions in Table 3. Raw values are mean monthly insurer costs from the underlying data without adjustment

Figure 1. Derived Monthly Costs to Insurers.

4. DISCUSSION

Our results show that some insurers and some patients spend less on conventional prescription medications after enrollment in a MCP. Annualized, these cost savings equal $864.24 for insurers and $129.56 for patients, subject to the assumptions underlying our calculations. Monthly cannabis costs based on patient surveys are $141, slightly more than the cost savings experienced by insurers twelve months post-enrollment. Patients experience much smaller conventional prescription medication cost savings ($20 by the twelfth month) and thus pay significantly more for cannabis than they save through reducing their prescription costs. This suggests that the benefits of cannabis sufficiently outweigh those of conventional prescriptions, so that patients are willing to pay more for cannabis and voluntarily reduce their conventional prescription fills, despite the lack of any requirement by their doctor to do so. This result is particularly strong for opioid medications, despite their highly addictive quality, supporting results in the literature that cannabis may be a non-lethal, viable substitute for opioids in chronic pain populations [11-13, 15]. The results are also stronger for Medicaid and Commercial insurer costs relative than Medicare and workers compensation, suggesting that demographic factors likely are at play. For example, Medicare patients are retired and older, while workers compensation patients may be disproportionately in occupations that require random drug testing.

In order to contain the analysis and limit the number of assumptions, we did not include the costs of office visits required for prescription refills and MCP referral, treatment for prescription drug or medical cannabis abuse, or common policy-level (rather than drug-level) features of insurance policies (e.g., coinsurance, deductibles, out-of-pocket maximums). Opioids, for example, require office visits every three months to maintain a continuous supply, while medical cannabis eligibility in the MCP requires an annual referral. Given that insurers do not pay for cannabis referral appointments, any reduction in the number of office visits associated with prescription refills would be a cost savings. For patients, the costs of office visits associated with prescription medications must be weighed against those associated with MCP referral. Typical office visit copayments for patients range from $8 (Medicaid) to $45 (commercial insurance). Patients in our sample paid $200 out-of-pocket to their physician for their initial medical cannabis referral and any associated annual renewal visits. With typical conventional prescription renewal office visit copayments, patients would face between $32 and $180 out of pocket per year versus $200 for a medical cannabis referral visit, only increasing the gap between what patients pay for cannabis and what they pay for prescriptions.

In line with research showing providers prescribe opioid therapies (e.g., oxycodone) as their first choice of treatment for chronic pain [23], most prescriptions taken by patients in our sample were opioid medications (59%) with the second most common benzodiazepines (27%), both associated with significant abuse potential and risk of death [24]. Cannabis users also face risks of dependence and abuse, but without the risk of death [25, 26] associated with opioid and benzodiazepine medications. Insurers currently risk paying for cannabis abuse treatment; however, with therapy primarily consisting of behavioral approaches, the cost of treatment would be lower than treatments involving continued use of potentially dangerous prescription treatments such as buprenorphine and methadone [27-29]. In other words, any reduction in costs associated with abuse of opioids would increase the cost savings to insurers from policyholder MCP enrollment. For patients, should addictive behavior arise and require treatment, the number of copayments for opioid abuse treatment presumably is higher than for cannabis abuse treatment because opioid abuse treatment includes both behavioral and medication-based interventions, thus reducing the expected cost increase associated with adding cannabis to a patient's medication regimen.

Although patients covered by Medicaid and workers compensation do not generally face coinsurance rates, annual deductibles, and out-of-pocket maximums, other health insurers often include these product features. These features would serve to shift costs between insurers and patients, but are unlikely to affect overall shifts in costs from conventional prescriptions to cannabis. In addition, our results for Medicaid and commercial insurers are strongest, suggesting that the effect is common across insurance policies with and without these features.

Although most patients likely pay more out-of-pocket to obtain cannabis than pharmaceutical medications, some grow their own cannabis thus avoiding the costs of buying from dispensaries in exchange for the costs of growing cannabis oneself. These costs range from fairly low gardening-associated costs for those utilizing natural growing resources outdoors (e.g., seasonal sunlight and water) to several thousand dollars for elaborate indoor growing environments. Despite the possible savings, only 14% of patients in New Mexico obtain personal production licenses [30], perhaps because dispensary customers generally have access to a broader range of products. With estimated first year post-enrollment cost savings of $20, even home cultivation is more expensive to the average patient than continuing their conventional prescription medication use without adding medical cannabis.

Our study has limitations. Due to federal restrictions, we did not perform a randomized control trial [31]. Therefore, selection effects may be affecting our results. For example, patients may enroll in the MCP to reduce their dependence on prescription medications, while those who do not enroll may be experiencing fewer adverse effects from their prescription medications. Including only back pain patients from a single clinic improves the internal validity of the results, but limits their generalizability to other patient populations. We also are not able to measure consumption of non-scheduled prescription drugs or diversion. Cannabis access may induce a shift toward non-scheduled prescriptions leading us to overestimate the cost savings associated with MCP enrollment. Our sample size was also fairly small, although we had sufficient statistical power to generate robust estimates of the downward trend post-enrollment among the MCP patients. Another concern is that physician-directed prescription reduction drove our results. However, this hypothesis is not supported by increase in prescription costs during month 19, the month of the annual MCP renewal visit.

It is not clear that we are observing long-run cost tradeoffs. Cannabis prices have been falling nationwide as markets have expanded [32]. In New Mexico, the average price fell by $1 per gram with the licensing of 12 additional producers in 2015. (Supplemental Appendix Figure SA1). In addition, patients are purchasing much less than the legally permissible amount of cannabis, which may be optimal, but could be indicative of economic inefficiencies in the market, e.g., supply constraints such as legal limits on number of producers (35) and plants per producer (450) may have led to high prices through lack of competition and reduced economies of scale [33]. If growing markets continue to put downward pressure on prices, cannabis could eventually become a low-cost alternative to prescription medications currently covered by insurers.

Supplemental Appendix

Table SA1. Descriptive Statistics for Cost Measures Underlying Calculated Cost Outcomes

Variable	Obs	Mean	Std. Dev.	Min	Max	N Patients Affected
Monthly Pill Cost (AWP)	2228	$286.44	$480.50	$0.00	$4,754.80	94
Out-of-pocket	2228	$23.80	$133.38	$0.00	$2,361.60	28
Medicaid	2228	$23.00	$127.93	$0.00	$1,771.20	15
Medicare	2228	$23.43	$152.33	$0.00	$2,871.00	20
Commercial	2228	$158.05	$385.53	$0.00	$4,754.80	79
Workers Compensation	2228	$27.17	$135.37	$0.00	$2,403.90	42
Monthly Opioid Pill Costs	2228	$186.31	$381.82	$0.00	$4,754.40	75
Monthly Prescriptions Filled	2228	1.24	1.29	0.00	10.00	
Out-of-pocket	2228	0.11	0.41	0.00	4.00	
Medicaid	2228	0.06	0.31	0.00	4.00	
Medicare	2228	0.12	0.52	0.00	6.00	
Commercial	2228	0.60	0.97	0.00	7.00	
Workers Compensation	2228	0.15	0.53	0.00	6.00	
Monthly Opioid Prescriptions Filled	2228	0.74	0.84	0.00	6.00	
Age	2228	55.0	12.0	23.3	87.4	
Male	2228	0.66	0.47	0.00	1.00	

Notes: Data are patient-month level. Costs are aggregated across prescriptions by month and by type as specified. Monthly Pill Costs refers to multiplying the number of dosages by the Average Wholesale Price. Monthly Prescriptions Filled refers to the total number of prescriptions filled by in the average patient-month. Number of users refers to how many users reported overall monthly pill costs and then monthly pill costs by type of payer.

Table SA2. Comparing 1st Six Months across Groups and 1st v. Last for the Comparison Group

Panel A: First Six Months

	Comparison	MCP	P Value
Monthly Costs to Insurers	288.30	250.53	0.260
Monthly Opioid Costs to Insurers	197.87	186.54	0.688
Monthly Costs to Patients	69.41	71.08	0.882
Monthly Opioid Costs to Patients	37.26	17.50	0.018

Panel B: Comparison Only - First v. Last Six Months

	1st Six Months	Last Six Months	P Value
Monthly Costs to Insurers	288.30	282.23	0.847
Monthly Opioid Costs to Insurers	197.87	184.09	0.583
Monthly Costs to Patients	54.31	65.90	0.332
Monthly Opioid Costs to Patients	37.26	49.54	0.274

Notes: This table compares the MCP and comparison groups of patients during the first six months of observation in Panel A and during the last six months of observation in Panel B. P-values correspond to two-sided t-tests for continuous variables and chi-squared tests for dichotomous variables. Data are patient-month level. Costs to Insurers are calculated as 0.86*Monthly Costs (AWP)+3.65*Monthly Rx Filled, while Costs to Patients are calculated as out-of-pocket costs plus copays of $5 (Medicaid) and $40 (Medicare and Commercial) times the Number of Prescriptions Filled that were covered by each payer. AWP, Average Wholesale Price.

Table SA3. Results from Random Effects Regressions

	(1)	(2)	(3)	(4)
Outcome ($)	Monthly Costs to Insurers	Monthly Costs to Patients	Monthly Opioid Costs to Insurers	Monthly Opioid Costs to Patients
Trend 1 (Months 1-6)	-6.987	-0.445	-5.031	0.699
	(7.680)	(2.029)	(5.743)	(1.655)
MCP * Trend 1	11.40	2.275	2.318	-0.470
	(11.30)	(2.398)	(9.216)	(1.749)
Trend 2 (Months 7 to 24)	0.718	1.065	0.309	0.665
	(2.142)	(0.740)	(1.343)	(0.618)
MCP * Trend 2	-11.13***	-1.667*	-7.339***	-0.839
	(3.539)	(0.944)	(2.344)	(0.672)
MCP	-33.32	-10.52	-11.86	-27.83
	(71.55)	(24.45)	(53.16)	(18.55)
Age	-1.760	2.893	-2.635	0.263
	(17.31)	(2.763)	(10.88)	(1.800)
Age-Squared	-0.0109	-0.0307	0.0257	-0.0049
	(0.155)	(0.0245)	(0.101)	(0.0172)
Male	17.66	-3.686	18.69	-8.985
Outcome ($)	(1) Monthly Costs to Insurers	(2) Monthly Costs to Patients	(3) Monthly Opioid Costs to Insurers	(4) Monthly Opioid Costs to Patients
	(59.04)	(20.45)	(44.52)	(16.34)
Constant	401.6	-1.302	230.6	51.13
	(481.6)	(93.73)	(304.4)	(63.06)
Patient-Month Observations	2,228	2,228	2,228	2,228
Number of Patients	94	94	94	94

Notes: The regressions replicate the main (patient-level) fixed effects regressions in Table 3 using random effect generalized linear regression models. Each column represents a separate regression measuring the association between MCP enrollment and costs to insurers (0.86*Monthly Pill Costs + 3.65*Monthly Prescriptions Filled) in the first column, and costs to patients (Monthly Cut-of-Pocket Costs (AWP) + $5*Number of Medicaid Prescriptions Filled + $40 * (Number of Medicare and Commercial Prescriptions Filled)). The regressions in Columns (3) and (4) replicate the regressions in Columns (1) and (2) including only opioid prescription-related costs in the outcome variables. Trend 1 refers to a linear trend during months 1 to 6 and Trend 2 measures a linear trend in Months 7 to 24. MCP designates enrollment in the MCP program. The interactions between MCP and the linear trends measure the differential effect of the trend among the MCP patient group relative to the comparison group. Standard errors are clustered at the patient level and reported in parentheses below the coefficients. * p<0.01, **p<0.05, *** p<0.01.

Table SA4. Results from Random Effects Regressions by Payer Type – Insurer Costs

Payer	Medicaid	Medicare	Commercial	Workers Compensation
Trend 1 (Months 1-6)	1.622	0.681	-6.999	0.0159
	(1.858)	(0.513)	(7.089)	(1.940)
MCP * Trend 1	-3.953	0.840	10.80	0.169
	(2.527)	(3.709)	(10.39)	(2.105)
Trend 2 (Months 7 to 24)	-0.0004	-0.177	1.001	0.428
	(0.226)	(0.155)	(1.657)	(1.076)
MCP * Trend 2	-2.048**	0.205	-5.117*	-0.959
	(0.920)	(1.196)	(2.730)	(1.124)
MCP	13.80	20.38	-67.36	-34.46**
	(18.96)	(17.14)	(61.50)	(17.18)
Age	1.071	5.678*	-16.04	3.415
	(3.632)	(3.196)	(14.69)	(2.868)
Age-Squared	-0.0096	-0.0523*	0.123	-0.0347
	(0.0306)	(0.0295)	(0.133)	(0.0230)
Male	-27.09	33.90**	13.56	7.098
	(20.96)	(16.69)	(48.21)	(15.45)
Constant	8.002	-158.0*	669.3*	-39.18
	(99.96)	(90.80)	(404.4)	(89.25)
Patient-Month Observations	2,228	2,228	2,228	2,228
Number of Patients	94	94	94	94

Notes: The regressions replicate the fixed effects regressions by for prescription costs regressions by each payer in Table 4 using random effect generalized linear regression models. Each column represents costs for a different payer as specified in the column title. The outcome is payer-specific costs, calculated as 0.86*Monthly Pill Costs + 3.65*Monthly Prescriptions Filled. Trend 1 refers to a linear trend during months 1 to 6 and Trend 2 measures a linear trend in Months 7 to 24. MCP designates enrollment in the MCP program. The interactions between MCP and the linear trends measure the differential effect of the trend among the MCP patient group relative to the comparison group. Standard errors are clustered at the patient level and reported in parentheses below the coefficients. * p<0.01, **p<0.05, *** p<0.01.

Table SA5: Results from Random Effects Regression by Payer – Patient Costs

Payer	Patient Out-of-Pocket	Medicaid	Medicare	Commercial
Trend 1 (Months 1-6)	-2.892	0.0826	4.761	-11.46
	(23.32)	(0.233)	(3.724)	(7.093)
MCP * Trend 1	0.0800	-0.0090	0.207	-0.723
	(2.015)	(0.0557)	(0.148)	(0.778)
Trend 2 (Months 7 to 24)	0.584	-0.0671	0.722	1.256
	(2.222)	(0.0678)	(0.468)	(1.159)
MCP * Trend 2	0.756	-0.0001	-0.0181	0.327
	(0.702)	(0.0066)	(0.0362)	(0.285)
MCP	-0.957	-0.0233*	-0.0226	-0.891**
	(0.813)	(0.0130)	(0.170)	(0.426)
Age	3.273	0.0250	1.117**	-1.611
	(2.030)	(0.0485)	(0.486)	(1.505)
Age-Squared	-0.0330*	-0.0002	-0.0101**	0.0136
	(0.0170)	(0.0004)	(0.0044)	(0.0142)
Male	-3.301	-0.301	7.327**	-7.928
	(19.96)	(0.256)	(2.936)	(5.664)
Constant	-48.98	-0.138	-31.48**	81.75**
	(78.84)	(1.349)	(14.20)	(40.64)
Patient-Month Observations	2,228	2,256	2,256	2,256
Number of Patients	94	94	94	94

Notes: The regressions replicate the fixed effects regressions by for patient costs associated with prescriptions covered by each payer individually in Table 4 using random effect generalized linear regression models. Each column represents a separate regression for prescription costs associated with each payer type. Insurer-specific costs are measured at the AWP. Patient out-of-pocket costs are measured as the number of prescriptions covered by that insurer times the associated copay, $5 for Medicaid and $40 for Medicare and Commercial insurance. Trend 1 refers to a linear trend during months 1 to 6 and Trend 2 measures a linear trend in Months 7 to 24. MCP designates enrollment in the MCP program. The interactions between MCP and the linear trends measure the differential effect of the trend among the MCP patient group relative to the comparison group. Standard errors are clustered at the patient level and reported in parentheses below the coefficients. * p<0.01, ** p<0.05, *** p<0.01.

Table SA6. Results from Regressions Omitting Patients with Censored Observation Periods

Outcome ($)	(1) Monthly Costs to Insurers	(2) Monthly Costs to Patients	(3) Monthly Opioid Costs to Insurers	(4) Monthly Opioid Costs to Patients
Trend 1 (Months 1-6)	-6.987	-0.445	-5.031	0.699
	(7.686)	(2.030)	(5.747)	(1.658)
MCP * Trend 1	1.397	2.897	-6.336	-1.089
	(12.15)	(2.369)	(11.03)	(1.766)
Trend 2 (Months 7 to 24)	0.718	1.065	0.309	0.665
	(2.143)	(0.740)	(1.344)	(0.619)
MCP * Trend 2	-11.28***	-0.740	-7.112***	-0.403
	(4.103)	(0.950)	(2.351)	(0.683)
MCP				-35.11
				(19.34)
Age				-0.287
				(1.935)
Age-Squared				0.000
				(0.017)
Male				-14.99
				(20.62)
Constant	250.2***	46.50***	160.5***	69.75
	(13.96)	(3.575)	(8.476)	(76.29)
Patient-Month Observations	1,800	1,800	1,800	1,800
R-Squared - Within	0.026	0.003	0.022	
Number of Patients	75	75	75	75

Notes: The regressions replicate the main regressions in Table 3 including only patients without censored observation periods. Each column represents a separate regression measuring the association between MCP enrollment and costs to insurers (0.86*Monthly Pill Costs + 3.65*Monthly Prescriptions Filled) in the first column, and costs to patients (Monthly Out-of-Pocket Costs (AWP) + $5*Number of Medicaid Prescriptions Filled + $40 * (Number of Medicare and Commercial Prescriptions Filled)). The regressions in Columns (3) and (4) replicate the regressions in Columns (1) and (2) including only opioid prescription-related costs in the outcome variables. Trend 1 refers to a linear trend during months 1 to 6 and Trend 2 measures a linear trend in Months 7 to 24. MCP designates enrollment in the MCP program. The interactions between MCP and the linear trends measure the differential effect of the trend among the MCP patient group relative to the comparison group. Individual patient fixed effects are included in a ordinary least squares panel regression model and the within-patient R-squareds are reported, i.e., the explanatory effect of the patient fixed effects is conditioned out prior to estimation of the main effects. Standard errors are clustered at the patient level and reported in parentheses below the coefficients. * p<0.01, ** p<0.05, *** p<0.01.

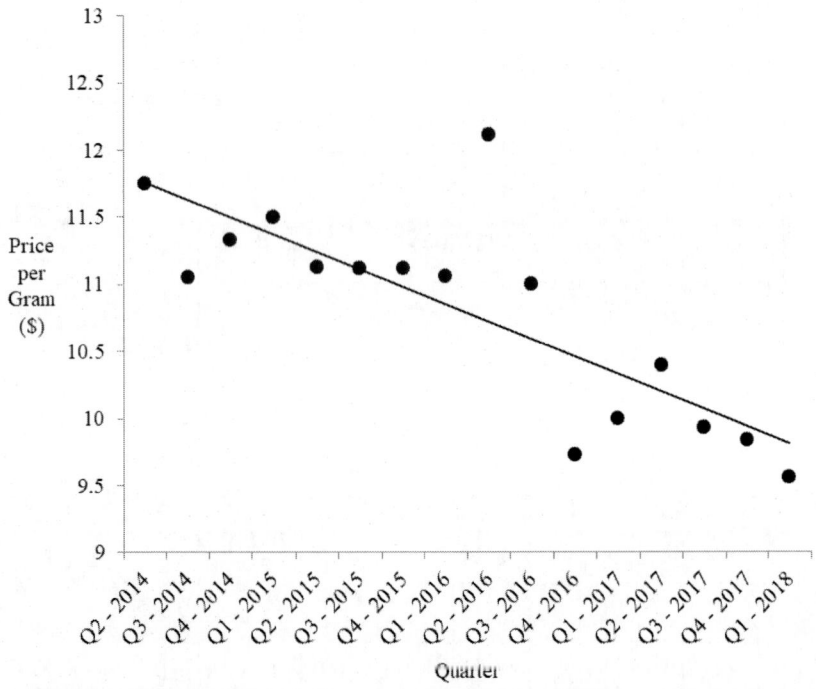

Notes: Each quarter, the New Mexico Medical Cannabis Program posts average per gram prices for flower sold in the state. These are available at https://nmhealth.org/about/mcp/svcs/pdb/. (Accessed 06/28/2018.) A linear trend is estimated based on the monthly prices.

Figure SA1. New Mexico Cannabis Prices by Quarter.

REFERENCES

[1] Gaskin, D. J., & Richard, P. (2012). The economic costs of pain in the United States. *Journal of Pain, 13(8)*, 715-724. doi: 10.1016/j.jpain.2012.03.009.

[2] Kane-Gill S. L., Rubin E. C., Smithburger P. L., Buckley M. S., & Dasta J. F. (2014).The cost of opioid-related adverse drug events. *Journal of Pain and Palliative Care Pharmacotherapy 28(3)*, 282–293. doi: 10.3109/15360288.2014.938889.

[3] Gilson, A. M., & Kreis P. G. (2009). The burden of the nonmedical use of prescription opioid analgesics. *Pain Medicine, 10(2)*, S89–S100. doi: 10.1111/j.1526-4637.2009.00668.x.

[4] Strassels S. A. (2009). Economic burden of prescription opioid misuse and abuse. *Journal of Managed Care & Specialty Pharmacy, 15(7)*, 556–62. doi: 10.18553/jmcp.2009.15.7.556.

[5] Centers for Disease Control. (2016). Wide-ranging online data for epidemiologic research (WONDER). Atlanta, GA: CDC, National Center for Health Statistics; 2016. Available at http://wonder.cdc.gov.

[6] Rudd R. A., Seth P., David F., & Scholl L. (2016). Increases in drug and opioid-involved overdose deaths—United States, 2010-2015. *Morbidity and Mortalilty Weekly Report*, 65, 1445-1452. doi: 10.15585/mmwr.mm655051e1.

[7] Taylor R., Pergolizzi J. V., Puenpatom R. A., & Summers K. H. (2013). Economic implications of potential drug–drug interactions in chronic pain patients. *Expert Review of Pharmacoeconomics & Outcomes Research, 13(6)*, 725-734. doi: 10.1586/14737167.2013.851006.

[8] Bradford, A. C., & Bradford, W. D. (2016). Medical marijuana laws reduce prescription medication use in Medicare Part D. *Health Affairs, 35(7)*, 1230-1236. doi: 10.1377/hlthaff.2015.1661.

[9] Bradford, A. C., & Bradford, W. D. (2017). Medical marijuana laws may be associated with a decline in the number of prescriptions for Medicaid Enrollees. *Health Affairs, 36(5)*, 945-951. doi: 10.1377/hlthaff.2016.1135.

[10] Bachhuber, M. A.; Saloner, B.; Cunningham, C. O., & Barry, C. L. (2014). Medical cannabis laws and opioid analgesic overdose mortality in the United States, 1999-2010. *JAMA Internal Medicine, 174(10)*, 1668-1673. doi: 10.1001/jamainternmed.2014.4005.

[11] Powell, David, Rosalie L. Pacula, and Mireille Jacobson. 2018. Do medical marijuana laws reduce addictions and deaths related to pain killers? *Journal of Health Economics*, 58, 29-42. doi.org/10.1016/j.jhealeco.2017.12.007.

[12] Wen, Hefei, and Jason M. Hockenberry. 2018. Association of Medical and Adult-Use Marijuana Laws With Opioid Prescribing for Medicaid Enrollees. *JAMA Internal Medicine, 178(5),* 673-679. doi:10.1001/jamainternmed.2018.1007.

[13] Vigil, J. M., Stith, S. S., Adams, I. M., & Reeve, A. P. (2017). Associations between medical cannabis and prescription opioid use in chronic pain patients: A preliminary cohort study. *PLoS ONE.* 12(11): e0187795. doi: 10.1371/journal.pone.0187795.

[14] Stith, S. S., Vigil, J. M., Adams, I. M., & Reeve, A. P. (2017). Effects of legal access to cannabis on Scheduled II-V Drug Prescriptions. *Journal of the American Medical Directors Association, 19(1),* 59-64. doi: 10.1016/j.jamda.2017.07.017.

[15] Haroutounian, S.; Ratz, Y.; Ginosar, Y.; Furmanov, K.; Saifi, F.; Meidan, R.; & Davidson, E. The effect of medicinal cannabis on pain and quality-of-life outcomes in chronic pain: A prospective open-label study. *Clinical Journal of Pain, 32(12),*1036-1043. doi: 10.1097/AJP.0000000000000364.

[16] Piper, B. J.; DeKeuster, R. M.; Beals, M. L.; Cobb, C. M.; Burchman, C. A.; Perkinson, L.; Lynn, S. T.; Nichols, S. D.; & Abess, A.T. (2017). *Substitution of medical cannabis for pharmaceutical agents for pain, anxiety, and sleep. Journal of Psychopharmacology, 31,* 569–575. doi: 10.1177/0269881117699616.

[17] *Truven Health Analytics.* (2017). Retrieved from https://truvenhealth.com/Portals/1/Assets/AWP%20Policy_Oct%202014.pdf.

[18] Sorenson A. T. (2000). Equilibrium price dispersion in retail markets for prescription drugs. *Journal of Political Economy,* 108(4), 833-850. doi: 10.1086/316103.

[19] Congressional Budget Office, The Congress of the United States (2007). Prescription Drug Pricing in the Private Sector. *A Congressional Budget Office Paper, January 2007,* 1-26.

[20] *Centers for Medicare and Medicaid Services.* (2018). Retrieved from https:// www.medicaid.gov/ medicaid-chip-program-information/ by-

topics/ prescription-drugs/ downloads/ xxxreimbursement-chart-current-qtr.pdf.
[21] *Kaiser Family Foundation.* (2016). Retrieved from https://www.kff.org/health-costs/report/2016-employer-health-benefits-survey/.
[22] *Centers for Medicare and Medicaid Services.* (2018). Medicare.gov Retrieved from https://www.medicare.gov/your-medicare-costs/costs-at-a-glance/costs-at-glance.html.
[23] Poulson, K. K., Andersen S. E., Moreno, S. I., Glintborg, D., Thirstrup. S., & Aagaard, L. (2013). General practitioners' and hospital physicians' preference for morphine or oxycodone as first-time choice for a strong opioid: a National Register-based study. *Basic & Clinical Pharmacology & Toxicology, 112(2),* 110-5. doi: 10.1111/j.1742-7843.2012.00927.x.
[24] Manchikanti, L., Helm, S. II, Fellows, B., Janata, J. W., Pampati, V., Grider, J. S., &Boswell, M. V. (2012). The Opioid Epidemic in the United States. *Pain Physician. 15(3 Suppl),*es9–es38.
[25] Calabria, B., Degenhardt, L., Hall, W., & Lynskey, M. (2010). Does cannabis use increase the risk of death? Systematic review of epidemiological evidence on adverse effects of cannabis use. *Drug and Alcohol Review, 29(3),* 318–30. doi: 10.1111/j.1465-3362.2009.00149.x.
[26] Fuster, D., Sanvisens, A., Bolao, F., Zuluaga, P., Rivas, I., Farre, M, Tor, J., & Muga, R. (2016). Cannabis as a secondary drug is not associated with a greater risk of death in patients with opiate, cocaine, or alcohol dependence. *Journal of Addiction Medicine, 11(1),* 34-39. doi: 10.1097/ADM.0000000000000266.
[27] Crane, E. H. (2013). *Emergency department visits involving buprenorphine.* The CBHSQ Report: January 29, 2013. Center for Behavioral Health Statistics and Quality, Substance Abuse and Mental Health Services Administration, Rockville, MD.
[28] Garcia-Portilla, M. P., Bobes-Bascaran, M. T., Bascaran, M. T., Saiz, P.A., & Bobes, J. (2012). Long term outcomes of pharmacological treatments for opioid dependence: does methadone still lead the pack?

British Journal of Clinical Pharmacology, 77, 272-284. doi: 10.1111/bcp.12031.

[29] Schuckit, M. A. (2016). Treatment of opioid-use disorders. *The New England Journal of Medicine, 375*, 357-368. doi: 10.1056/NEJMra1604339.

[30] New Mexico Department of Health (2017a). *Medical Cannabis Program Patient Statistics* – December 2017. Retrieved from https://nmhealth.org/publication/view/report/4174/.

[31] Stith, S. S., & Vigil, J. M. (2016). Federal barriers to Cannabis research. *Science, 352 (6290)*, 1182. doi: 10.1126/science.aaf7450.

[32] *Cannabis Benchmarks*. (2017, April 28). Retrieved from http://www.cannabisbenchmarks.com/uploads/5/0/4/5/50458953/twoyearchartfrom04.28.17forweb.pdf.

[33] New Mexico Department of Health. (2017b). *Medical Cannabis Licensed Non-Profit Producer Re-Licensures List for 2016/2017*. Retrieved from https://nmhealth.org/publication/view/general/2239/.

INDEX

A

abuse, 45, 64, 85, 95
acceptance, vii, viii, 8, 28, 42, 45, 46, 47, 55, 57, 59, 61, 65, 70
access, 19, 29, 31, 63, 65, 75, 77, 86, 87, 96
acupuncture, 23, 28, 40
adaptation, 28, 29, 43, 48
adaptations, 3, 44
adjustment, 47, 56, 84
adults, 24, 29, 48, 56
adverse effects, 63, 65, 87, 97
age, 2, 32, 50, 51
analgesic, 13, 14, 16, 18, 23, 95
anger, 12, 17
anxiety, 2, 3, 5, 7, 8, 10, 12, 13, 15, 24, 45, 55, 65, 68, 69, 96
arousal, 5, 12
assessment, 48, 49, 62
attitudes, 29, 50
autonomy, 49, 63
avoidance, 46, 65
awareness, 9, 49

B

back pain, vii, x, 14, 17, 24, 74, 76, 87
barriers, 33, 98
base, 45, 49, 65, 68, 69
behavior therapy, 46, 48
benefits, 47, 75, 84, 97
biofeedback, 22, 24
bio-psychosocial model, 29
bottom-up, 31, 38
brain, 2, 4, 13, 22, 65
breathing, 5, 7, 9

C

cancer, 2, 3, 19, 39, 43, 55, 56, 67
cannabis, v, vii, ix, 73, 74, 75, 76, 77, 78, 79, 81, 82, 83, 84, 85, 86, 87, 94, 95, 96, 97, 98
challenges, 47, 66
chronic illness, 28, 49
chronic illness and disease, 28
chronic pain, v, vii, viii, ix, 1, 2, 3, 4, 5, 6, 7, 8, 11, 12, 13, 16, 18, 19, 20, 21, 22, 23, 25, 27, 28, 29, 31, 32, 37, 38, 41, 44,

45, 48, 49, 53, 54, 55, 56, 57, 60, 61, 62, 63, 65, 67, 68, 70, 71, 74, 75, 85, 95, 96
clients, 24, 49, 53
coding, 35, 36, 37
commercial, 77, 79, 82, 85, 86
communication, viii, 1, 62
comparative method, 37, 52
compensation, 75, 77, 85, 86
complexity, 4, 28, 29, 50
construction, 37, 46, 50
constructivist approach, 31, 51
coping, v, viii, 11, 27, 28, 29, 30, 31, 34, 37, 39, 40, 41, 42, 43, 44, 45, 46, 47, 48, 49, 50, 51, 54, 55, 56, 64
coping strategies, 29, 39, 40, 46, 48, 49, 50, 51, 52, 55
cost, ix, 19, 74, 75, 76, 77, 79, 80, 81, 84, 85, 86, 87, 94
cost saving, ix, 74, 75, 76, 84, 85, 86, 87
creativity, 7, 25, 66
culture, 29, 38, 47
cure, 7, 17, 41, 45

D

data analysis, 31, 36
data collection, 33, 34, 36, 37, 50
database, ix, 60, 61
deaths, 75, 95
depression, 2, 3, 6, 7, 8, 13, 15, 20, 21, 29, 45, 48, 55, 65, 69
depth, 8, 30, 31, 35, 51
diet, 20, 40
disability, 46, 50
discomfort, 4, 14, 15
distress, vii, ix, 1, 47, 51, 60, 61
drawing, 8, 36
drug therapy, ix, 60, 61

E

education, 3, 61, 76
emotion, 11, 45
emotional distress, vii, viii, 1, 3, 18
emotional state, 2, 4, 8
empowerment, ix, 60, 61, 62, 63, 64
enduring, 28, 46, 51
enrollment, x, 74, 75, 76, 79, 80, 82, 84, 86, 87, 90, 91, 92, 93
evidence, viii, 2, 13, 19, 65, 76, 97
exercise, 7, 8, 17
exertion, 39, 40
expertise, 19, 24, 38
external locus of control, 45, 48

F

family members, 43, 47
fear, 5, 11, 46, 47, 62, 64, 65
feelings, vii, 1, 3, 5, 7, 8, 11, 13, 17, 38, 42, 48, 63
fibromyalgia, 13, 17, 20, 36, 55, 65
flexibility, 34, 65
fluid, 14, 15
fMRI, 20, 24
force, 39, 46

G

God, viii, 28, 41, 47
grounded theory, vii, viii, 27, 31, 34, 35, 38, 43, 50, 53, 54, 56

H

headache, 18, 32
healing, 14, 16, 54, 66
health, vii, viii, 1, 17, 29, 37, 42, 45, 49, 55, 56, 74, 86, 97

health care, vii, viii, 1, 29, 42, 49
health care professionals, 42, 49
health insurance, 74
health locus of control, 45, 55
history, 30, 49
HIV, 65, 68
human, 23, 28, 31, 50
hypnosis, viii, 2, 5, 6, 7, 8, 9, 10, 11, 12, 13, 14, 15, 16, 17, 18, 19, 20, 21, 22, 23, 24, 25, 65, 70

I

identification, 17, 34
identity, vii, 1, 3, 30, 45
image, 5, 6, 7, 9, 11, 14
imagery, viii, 2, 5, 7, 11, 13, 14, 16, 17, 18, 39, 45
imagination, viii, 1, 6, 7, 9, 11, 12, 18
individuals, 22, 29, 31, 39, 44, 46, 47, 48, 49, 50
induction, 9, 12, 22, 24
inflammation, 15, 32
injury, iv, 2, 22, 74
interdisciplinary pain management, 60
interference, vii, ix, 38, 60, 61, 62
intervention, 19, 54
interventions, v, 1, 19, 20, 21, 24, 25, 45, 49, 63, 64, 69, 86
islands, 28, 30
issues, 30, 42

L

light, viii, 2, 14, 28, 29, 44, 49, 50, 51
linear model, 46, 56
locus, 45, 48
lying, 12, 18

M

majority, 19, 51, 79
Maltese, v, vii, viii, 27, 28, 29, 32, 33, 38, 44, 47, 50, 51
management, vii, viii, 1, 3, 7, 11, 16, 18, 19, 25, 60, 61, 76
marijuana, 74, 75, 95, 96
MCP, x, 74, 75, 76, 77, 79, 80, 81, 82, 83, 84, 85, 86, 87, 89, 90, 91, 92, 93
Medicaid, 75, 77, 78, 79, 80, 82, 83, 85, 86, 88, 89, 90, 91, 92, 93, 95, 96, 97
medical, ix, 4, 28, 48, 53, 60, 61, 62, 74, 75, 76, 85, 86, 95, 96
Medicare, 75, 77, 78, 79, 80, 83, 85, 88, 89, 90, 91, 92, 93, 95, 96, 97
medication, x, 16, 18, 28, 44, 63, 64, 74, 76, 84, 86, 95
medicine, 54, 65
Merleau-Ponty, ix, 60, 61, 66
meta-analysis, 20, 21, 23
metaphor, 5, 15
methadone, 86, 97
methodology, vii, viii, 27, 31, 34, 38
Mexico, vii, x, 73, 74, 76, 77, 78, 79, 81, 82, 83, 84, 86, 87, 94, 98
mindfulness, v, ix, 49, 59, 60, 61, 64, 65, 68, 69, 70
misuse, 74, 95
models, 29, 80
mortality, 3, 95
motivation, 7, 19, 49, 63
multiple sclerosis, 6, 13, 22
musculoskeletal, 2, 55

N

narratives, 34, 37, 38
National Academy of Sciences, 21, 23
nationality, 32, 50

nerve, 28, 32, 40
neuralgia, 15, 17
neuroscience, viii, 2
neutral, 32, 34, 37

O

opioid, 24, 64, 67, 74, 75, 78, 79, 80, 81, 82, 85, 88, 89, 90, 93, 94, 95, 96, 97, 98

P

pain, v, vii, viii, ix, x, 1, 2, 3, 4, 5, 6, 7, 8, 11, 12, 13, 14, 15, 16, 17, 18, 19, 20, 21, 22, 23, 24, 27, 28, 29, 30, 31, 32, 33, 34, 36, 37, 38, 39, 40, 41, 42, 43, 44, 45, 46, 47, 48, 49, 50, 51, 52, 53, 54, 55, 56, 57, 59, 60, 61, 62, 63, 64, 65, 66, 67, 68, 69, 70, 71, 74, 75, 76, 85, 87, 94, 95, 96, 97
pain coping, vii, viii, 27, 29, 30, 31, 34, 44, 46, 50, 51, 52
pain management, vii, viii, ix, 13, 22, 28, 33, 49, 50, 54, 56, 59, 60, 61, 62, 66, 70, 71
participants, vii, viii, 27, 30, 31, 32, 33, 34, 35, 36, 37, 38, 40, 41, 42, 45, 47, 50, 51
pharmaceutical, ix, 60, 61, 62, 75, 86, 96
pharmacoeconomic, 74, 95
pharmacological treatment, 39, 51, 97
physical activity, 10, 64
physicians, 64, 97
population, 2, 21, 29, 30, 50
positive suggestion, 2, 8
prescription costs, 77, 79, 80, 83, 84, 87, 91, 92
prescription drugs, 87, 96
preservation, viii, 28, 39, 45
professionals, 5, 8, 18, 19, 48, 49
psychological, v, viii, ix, 1, 2, 18, 20, 21, 23, 24, 25, 28, 29, 31, 33, 34, 37, 42, 45, 47, 48, 49, 50, 52, 53, 55, 56, 59, 60, 65, 69, 70
psychological distress, viii, 2, 48
psychological well-being, 48, 53
psychology, 17, 33
P-value, 81, 89

Q

qualitative research, 35, 53, 54
quality of life, 28, 29, 49, 50, 63

R

reality, 18, 23, 44, 51
recommendations, iv, 35, 49
reflexivity, 31, 54
regression, x, 74, 76, 79, 80, 82, 83, 90, 91, 92, 93
regression model, 79, 90, 91, 92, 93
relaxation, 5, 8, 9, 10, 13, 20, 21, 22, 39
relief, 4, 7, 12, 14, 40
religion, viii, 27, 30, 47
researchers, 30, 31, 50
resistance, 45, 49
resources, vii, viii, 1, 65, 86
response, 2, 5, 12, 15
restructuring, 22, 45, 62
risk, 38, 46, 48, 56, 63, 64, 74, 85, 97

S

savings, x, 74, 84, 86
self-efficacy, v, vii, ix, 46, 47, 50, 53, 59, 60, 61, 62, 64, 65, 68
self-empowerment, v, ix, 59, 60, 61, 62, 63, 64
sensation, 2, 16
sensations, 3, 15, 47
senses, 9, 10, 12

sensitivity, 36, 83
services, iv, 28, 29, 31, 32, 49, 50
shock, 4, 17
showing, 14, 85
side effects, viii, 1, 74, 75
smoking, 25, 40
social support, 41, 45, 46, 48, 65
society, 41, 43, 51
solution, viii, 24, 27, 43, 47, 53, 54, 66
spirituality, 45, 46, 55
standard error, 82, 83
state, 5, 6, 8, 9, 10, 12, 15, 18, 75, 94
states, 62, 64
statistics, 46, 79
stimulation, 28, 40
stress, 3, 12, 17, 24, 31
suicidal ideation, 46, 48
suicide, viii, 27, 43, 46, 47, 48, 54, 57
Switzerland, 59, 71
symptoms, vii, 1, 4, 6, 11, 45, 46

T

techniques, viii, ix, 2, 8, 9, 13, 14, 19, 24, 45, 46, 47, 60, 61, 65

temperature, 10, 14
temporomandibular disorders, 13, 20
therapeutic interventions, 19, 49, 64
therapist, 48, 62
therapy, ix, 22, 24, 47, 48, 53, 54, 55, 60, 61, 62, 63, 64, 65, 68, 86
thoughts, 8, 11, 12, 36, 47, 48, 49
tissue, 2, 4
training, 17, 18, 19, 22, 24, 48
treatment, vii, ix, 5, 21, 22, 28, 34, 48, 49, 55, 60, 61, 63, 64, 65, 66, 75, 76, 85
trial, 23, 24, 55, 87

W

waking, 5, 9
walking, 3, 40
water, 12, 16, 86
wellness, 39, 45
wholesale, x, 74
workers, 75, 85, 86

Related Nova Publications

BEHAVIORAL STUDY OF 'NON-OPIOID TOLERANCE'

AUTHORS: Merab G. Tsagareli, Nana Tsiklauri (Ivane Beritashvili Institute of Physiology, Tbilisi, Georgia)

SERIES: Pain and its Origins, Diagnosis and Treatments

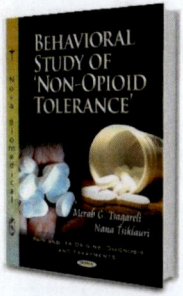

BOOK DESCRIPTION: Numerous anatomy-physiological studies have revealed a number of brain structures involved in the shaping of pain and endogenous analgesia. This book presents and examines current research discovered in a behavioral study of 'non-opioid' tolerance.

SOFTCOVER ISBN: 978-1-62100-033-4
RETAIL PRICE: $65

WHY 40%-80% OF CHRONIC PAIN PATIENTS ARE MISDIAGNOSED AND HOW TO CORRECT THAT

AUTHOR: Nelson H. Hendler, MD (Former Assistant Professor of Neurosurgery, Johns Hopkins University School of Medicine, Baltimore, MD, US)

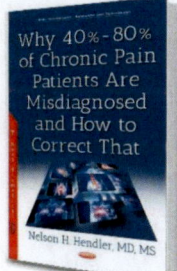

SERIES: Pain Management - Research and Technology

BOOK DESCRIPTION: The book addresses conceptual methods of problem solving, as they are applied to medicine. This book is designed to be the "Freakanomics" for medicine. Many research reports document that 40%-80% (or more, for certain disorders) of chronic pain patients are misdiagnosed. The leading causing of this failure is inadequate history taking, and the use of the wrong medical tests.

HARDCOVER ISBN: 978-1-53612-617-4
RETAIL PRICE: $230

Related Nova Publications

NAPROXEN: CHEMISTRY, CLINICAL ASPECTS AND EFFECTS

EDITOR: Judson Horner

SERIES: Pain Management – Research and Technology

BOOK DESCRIPTION: In *Naproxen: Chemistry, Clinical Aspects and Effects,* a compilation of the research developed in the past decades on synthetic receptors for naproxen is presented. Naproxen receptors proved their usefulness in chiral separation of the racemate and in other instances of supramolecular chemistry and pharmacy.

SOFTCOVER ISBN: 978-1-53614-129-0
RETAIL PRICE: $82

MANAGEMENT OF POSTOPERATIVE PAIN AFTER BARIATRIC SURGERY

EDITOR: Jaime Ruiz-Tovar, M.D., Ph.D. (Department of Surgery, Universidad Autónoma de Madrid, Spain)

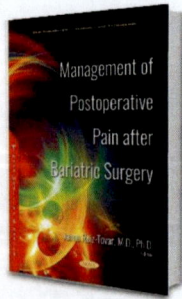

SERIES: Pain Management – Research and Technology

BOOK DESCRIPTION: Patients undergoing bariatric surgery are special subjects, as they present different conditions that make it more difficult to facilitate correct postoperative management. A medical staff is often not used to managing these patients and they do not consider that different measures or doses of drugs should be employed.

HARDCOVER ISBN: 978-1-53614-284-6
RETAIL PRICE: $95